Good
SKIN

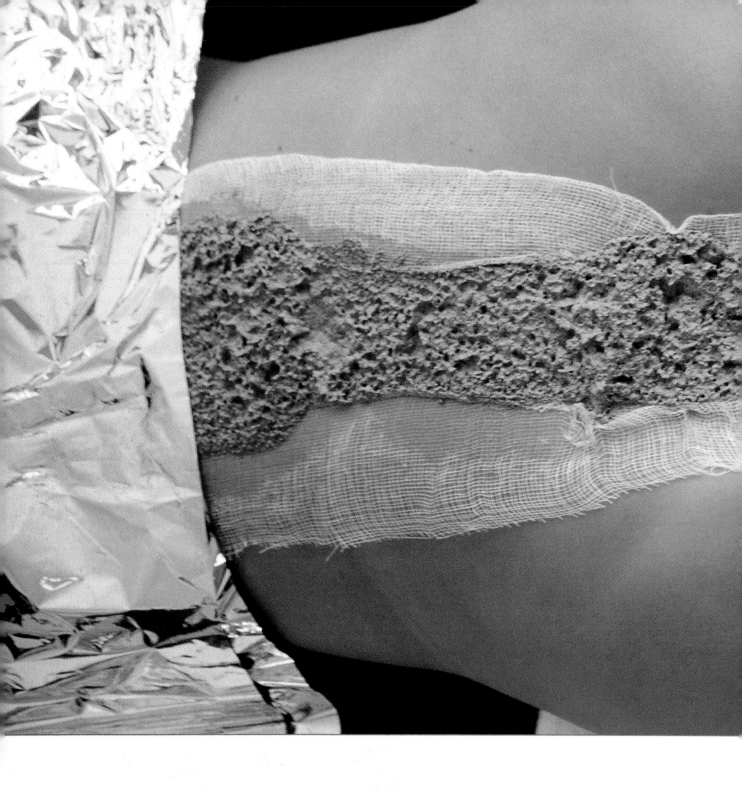

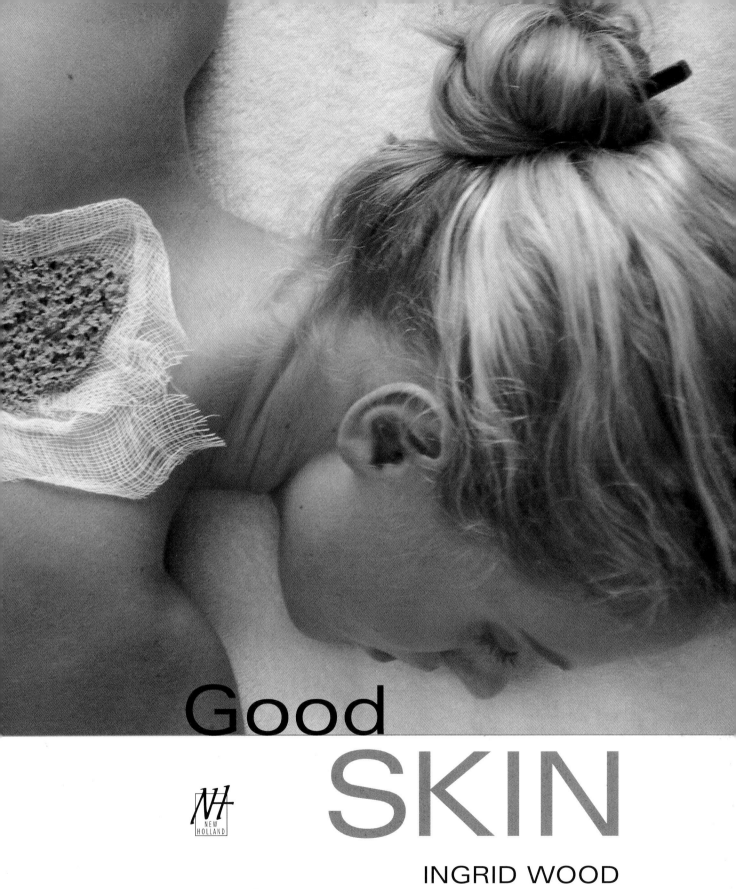

Good
SKIN

NEW HOLLAND

INGRID WOOD

First published in 2005 by
New Holland Publishers
London • Cape Town • Sydney • Auckland
www.newhollandpublishers.com

86 Edgware Rd
London W2 2EA
United Kingdom

80 McKenzie Street
Cape Town 8001
South Africa

14 Aquatic Drive
Frenchs Forest
NSW 2086
Australia

218 Lake Road
Northcote
Auckland
New Zealand

Publisher: Mariëlle Renssen
Publishing managers: Claudia dos Santos, Simon Pooley
Commissioning editor: Alfred LeMaitre
Studio manager: Richard MacArthur
Concept and design: Christelle Marais
Editor: Lauren Caplan
Illustrator: Alzette Prinz
Proofreader: Leizel Brown
Picture researchers: Karla Kik, Tamlyn McGeean
Production: Myrna Collins
Consultant: Beryl Barnard FSBTh. M.PHYS. ATT (Education
    Director, The London Schoolof Beauty & Make-up)

ISBN 1 84330 765 0 (HB); 1 84330 766 9 (PB)

Reproduction by Hirt & Carter (Cape) Pty Ltd
Printed and bound in Malaysia by Times Offset(M) Sdn. Bhd.

10 9 8 7 6 5 4 3 2

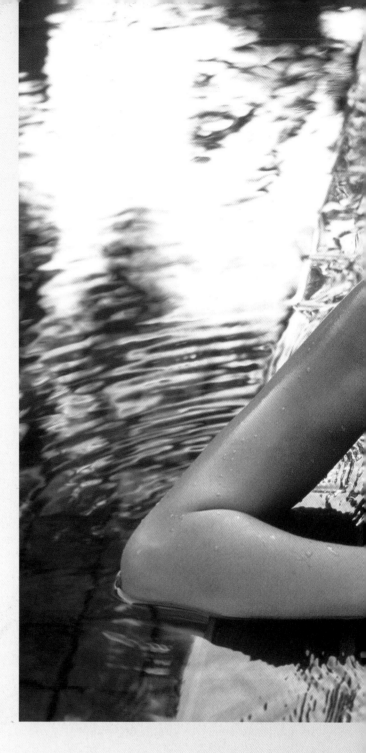

DISCLAIMER

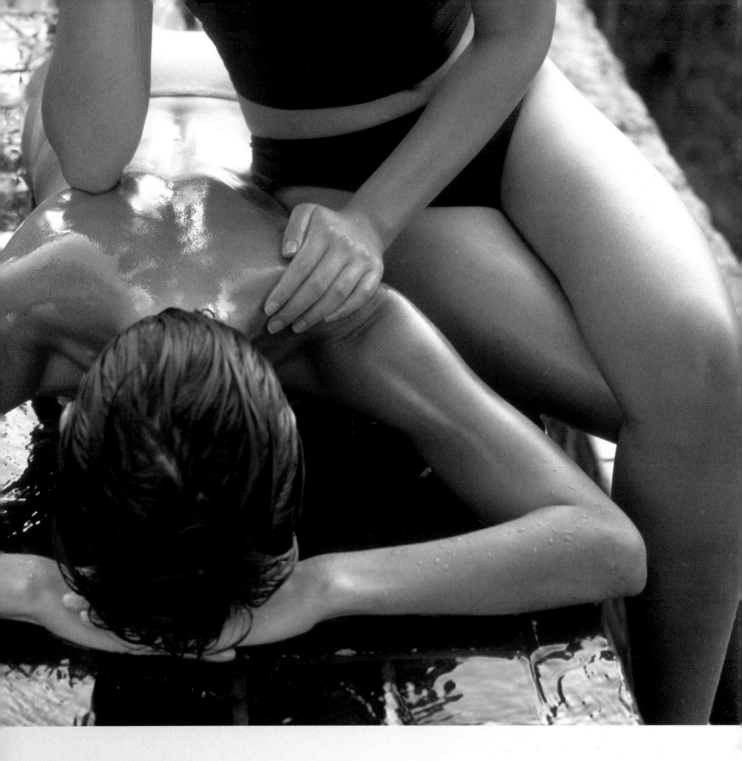

ACKNOWLEDGEMENTS
The publishers gratefully acknowledge the assistance of Ian Macfarlane from **MEDI-SPA** for the use of their beautiful
facilities during the photo shoot.
Medi-Spa: 99 Kloof Street, Gardens, Cape Town, 8001, South Africa
info@medispa.co.za; float@medispa.co.za; www.float.co.za

contents

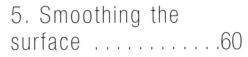

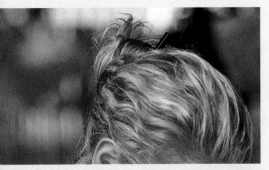

5. Smoothing the surface 60

Learn about rejuvenation techniques, from Botox and fillers to microdermabrasion, peels and laser treatment.

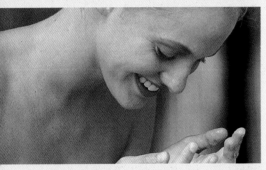

6. Taking care of your body . . .68

How to look after your body: correct diet, massage, posture and exercise, as well as procedures such as vein removal, and taking care of stretch marks.

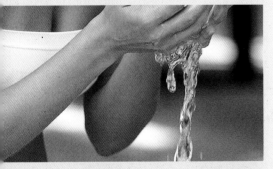

7. Feeding your skin 78

A closer look at how a healthy, balanced diet can prevent premature ageing, and various techniques that lower the effects of stress on the human body.

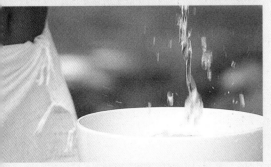

Unmasking skin

If you look in the mirror, your skin looks like a simple covering for the body. In fact this is a deceptive image: consider that the skin is the largest living organ in the human body, as essential and hard working as the brain or heart, and the closest contact we have with the outside world. It's literally our last outpost, and usually the unsung hero. Besides its obvious role of keeping our insides in, skin is also responsible for keeping foreign invaders out, regulating body temperature, getting rid of waste matter, acting as a water reservoir, manufacturing vitamin D from sunlight and housing our senses of touch and pain.

From a distance, your skin appears smooth and flat, but on closer inspection you will see that a network of tiny grooves, which change shape as the skin moves, marks the surface. A cross section looks a little like a complex Dagwood sandwich, with various layers and fillings. The two skin layers – the epidermis and dermis – rest on a third layer of subcutaneous fat, and send signals to the brain to set various physiological functions in motion. In order to take the best care of your skin, it's important to understand how these layers work.

Every day we shed about 4% of our total skin cells – that's about 14kg (30lb) in a lifetime.

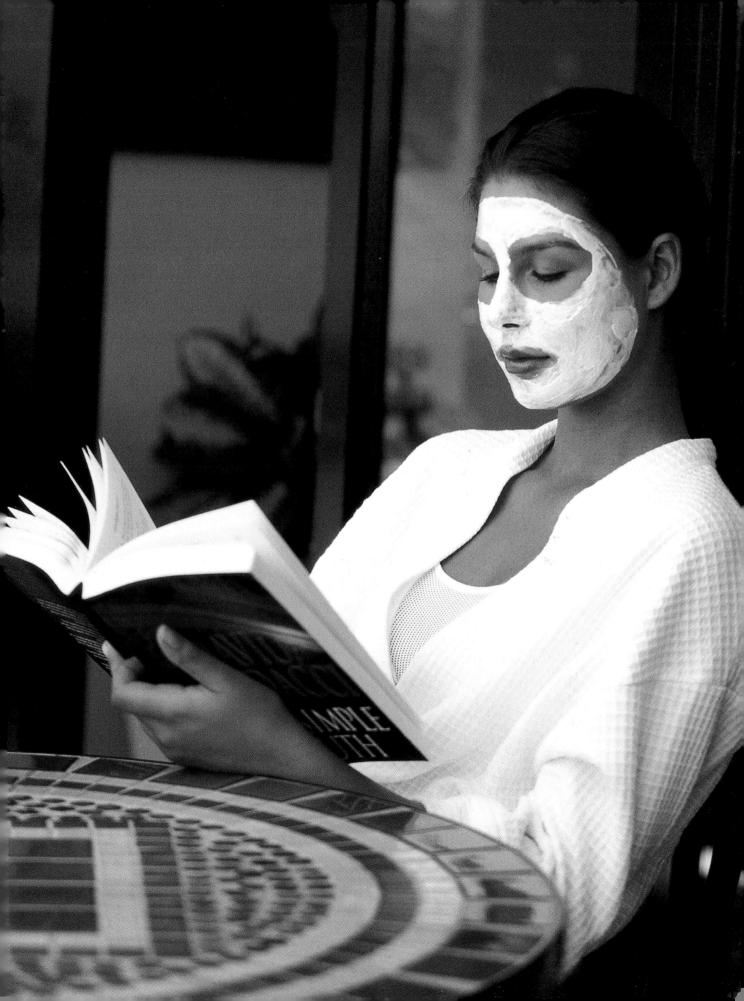

THE EPIDERMIS

Your skin's front line of defence is the epidermis. It allows light to partially pass through it as it would through frosted glass, and is nourished by blood vessels in the deeper layers of the skin that provide it with oxygen and 'skin food'. Plump, moist skin cells are developed in the basal layer of the epidermis. As each new layer of skin cells form, the cells move up towards the skin's surface, becoming flattened as they do so. By the time they reach the outer horny layer of the skin – known as the stratum corneum – they are effectively dead. These layers of densely packed cells, known as corneocytes, are filled with a protein called keratin, and a fatty lipid. Like the tiles of a roof, they overlap in layers to form a strong, protective shield that prevents water loss. Throughout your life, the cells of the surface layer are continually being worn away and replaced with new cells from below. In normal skin, it takes about 30 days for the cells to move up to the surface. If the outer layer is being lost quickly – due to sunburn, for example – these cells will be replaced more swiftly.

Below the stratum corneum are the Langerhans cells, which patrol for invaders, and the melanocytes – cells that produce the pigment melanin which helps determine the colour of your hair and skin. Melanocytes evolved to help the skin ward off dangerous UV radiation; the melanin on the skin surface absorbs UV light, protecting the cells below. Within the melanocyte, melanin is packaged in small membrane sacs called the melanosomes. The difference in pigmentation of various ethnic groups is due to the way in which the pigment is packed in these melanosomes. Skin cells in black-skinned people do not contain more melanocyte cells, but the melanin granules are larger and individually dispersed. Black-skinned people, therefore, are genetically programmed to be more resistant to UV damage because of the profusion of melanin within their cells. People with white skin tend to suffer more from unprotected sun exposure because they have less melanin, and because their melanosomes are smaller and grouped together in membrane-bound clumps. Skin cells in Asian people contain smaller

LAYERS OF THE SKIN

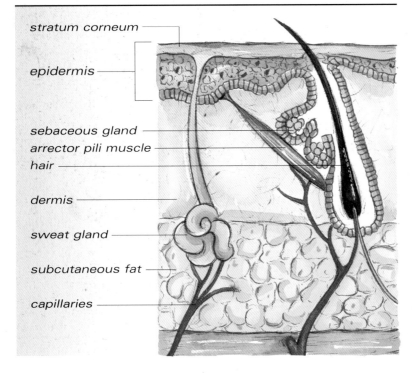

stratum corneum

epidermis

sebaceous gland

arrector pili muscle

hair

dermis

sweat gland

subcutaneous fat

capillaries

melanosome complexes that are more densely packed than those found in Caucasian skin cells.

THE DERMIS

The dermis is composed entirely of living cells. While the epidermis can repair itself, the dermis can become permanently damaged. This layer consists mainly of collagen, a protein that's responsible for the structural support (i.e. strength and resilience) of the skin. Collagen is packaged in bundles held together by elastic fibres. These are made up of another protein, elastin, which gives the skin its tone, plumpness and elasticity. Also found in the dermis are the sebaceous glands, hair follicles and sweat glands. The main function of sweat glands is to regulate the body's temperature. They are distributed over the entire body surface, with a larger number on the palms, soles and forehead. The sebaceous glands produce sebum (oil), the skin's natural lubricant. They are very sensitive to hormones, especially male hormones, which increase the glands' size and the secretion of sebum. (That's why males are more prone to acne, especially during puberty.) Sebaceous glands therefore play a key role in determining facial skin type.

MELANOSOME COMPLEXES

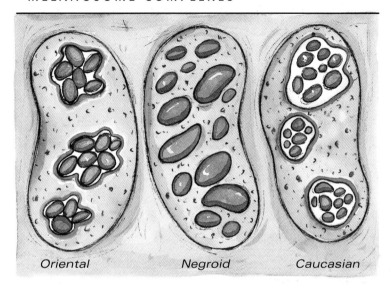

Oriental   Negroid   Caucasian

Do men and women age differently?

There is definitely a difference in male and female skin and so also in the ageing process. Women have less collagen than men to begin with, and because men have a thicker stratum corneum and produce more sebum than women, the lipid film on their skin surface is more pronounced. Furthermore, men's sebaceous glands are active well into their eighties. Also, testosterone, which is found in far higher levels in men, increases the rate of cell turnover in the basal layer and enhances collagen production, thereby thickening the skin. While there is a gradual thinning of skin with age in men (about 1% per year), the thickness of a woman's skin remains fairly consistent until menopause, when her oestrogen levels start to fall. Then she will experience a dramatic thinning of the skin, and decreased collagen synthesis and repair. In addition, there is an increase in intrinsic ageing with the failure of oestrogen production and reduced dermal hydration.

The functions of the skin

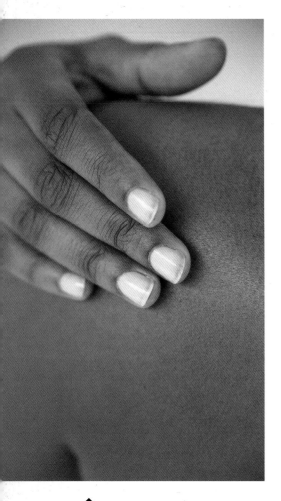

The concept of skincare is simple: be gentle. Treat it with tender loving care and it is going to reward you with a fresher and more youthful appearance later in life.

On one square inch of cheek there are some 30 nerves, 15 sensory receptors for cold, 80 receptors for heat and 1 300 pain receptors.

ABSORPTION AND ASSIMILATION

The skin is the gateway to the body and a barrier to the outside world. A substance can only be assimilated or used by the cells once it has been absorbed. Well-cleansed, exfoliated skin absorbs creams more easily, and massage or pressurized movements further aid this process. Absorption depends on the molecular structure of the product, which is why a moisturizer is absorbed, for example, but water and cleanser are not.

ELIMINATION

The skin rids the body of excess waste and toxins through the production of sweat and sebum.

SENSE OF TOUCH

The skin is full of nerve endings that transmit sensations like heat, cold, pressure and texture to the brain. Tingling skin, for example, is a neuro response and not an allergic response.

REGULATION OF BODY TEMPERATURE

The millions of veins, capillaries and arteries that traverse the skin, together with the sweat glands, regulate our internal body temperature so that it remains constant, regardless of the external temperature. This is made possible by the contraction and expansion of these vessels as necessary (in cold and in heat respectively), and the production of perspiration by the sweat glands to cool the body down when it overheats.

PROTECTION

The skin protects the body, both physically – from bumps, shocks and water loss – and chemically – from infection and dehydration – by means of the acid mantle.

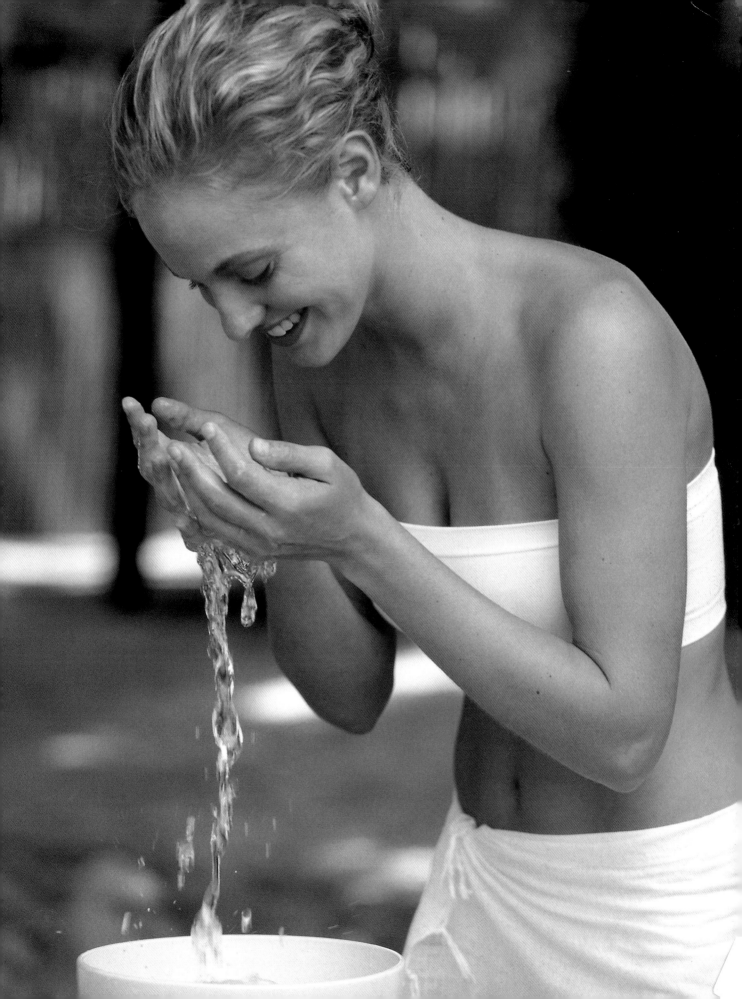

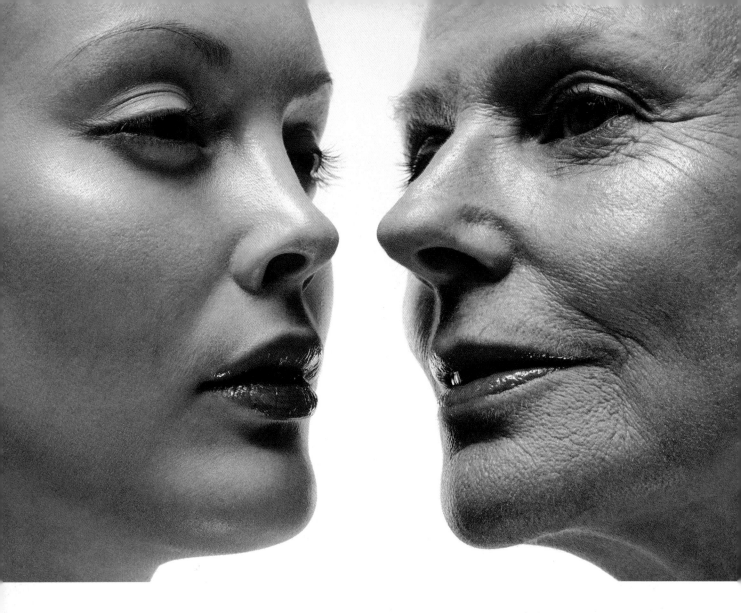

How skin ages

Your body is programmed to age and there's nothing you can do about your internal clock! The good news is there's a lot you can do to slow down the visible results of the process and keep your skin looking better for longer. There are two types of ageing – intrinsic and extrinsic.

Intrinsic or chronological ageing is the natural, biological process of ageing, over which we have little control. Extrinsic ageing is a result of external causes, in particular photo ageing (damage caused by ultra-violet radiation or sun exposure). Exposure to UV light and pollution

Genetics play an important role in determining how you will age. If your mother looked good well into her six-ties, chances are high you will too – if you look after yourself, of course.

accelerate ageing due to the production of free radicals in the skin. Free radicals are rogue molecules that attack the collagen and elastin fibres as well as new skin cells as they form. Although this happens mainly in the dermis, the effect is visible on the surface of the skin as a dry and weakened skin texture, pigmentation, broken veins and an increased vulnerability to further external damage.

The difference between intrinsic and extrinsic ageing can be seen on the inside of your upper arm, near the armpit. You will notice that this skin is smooth, soft and supple, while the skin on the back of the hands is thicker, rougher and drier. With intrinsic ageing, the skin's outer layer will become about 20% thinner over time, although the skin's surface should remain smooth. Sun-damaged skin, however, is thickened, with up to 50% more cells accumulating on the surface, giving it a rough, dry texture. (Think of a weather-beaten fisherman.) Photo ageing also causes a marked accumulation of pigment in the basal layers, resulting in age spots. In addition, pores tend to be more dilated and the skin may appear more mottled. And that's only the damage visible to the naked eye!

The thinnest skin is on the eyes, lips, neck and the back of the hands; and the thickest on the palms of the hands and soles of the feet.

Hands can give away age in a flash. Compared to the face, they have a thinner layer of skin, less fat to hide wrinkles, fewer oil glands to moisturize them and you can't use make-up to conceal them. The secret to good looking hands: take good care of them.

▼

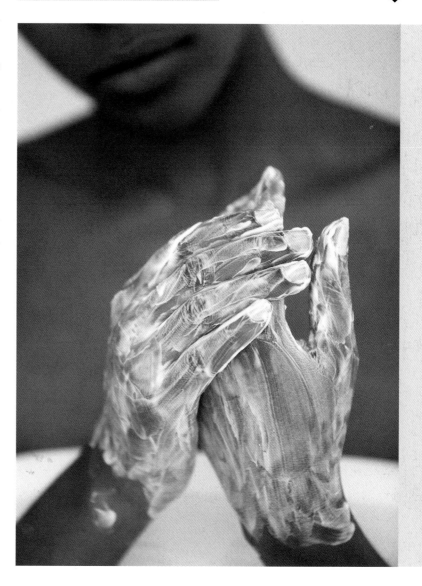

A lifetime of skin

Skin changes as we age. There is little you can do about it, but if you take good care of yourself throughout your lifetime, you can reduce the visible effects of the ageing process.

With age, the elasticity and strength of the skin declines. Coupled with the pull of gravity, this results in sagging and wrinkles. Although some products claim to 'restore' youth, there is nothing one can do to stop this decline. One can, however, preserve what one has by following a good care routine and minimizing sun exposure. It is mostly the damage done to deeper levels that determines how our skin looks as we get older, and this is largely self-inflicted by years of overexposure to the sun. Everyone's skin ages differently according to genetics, lifestyle choices, stress levels, exposure to things like ultraviolet light or harmful substances, and to a certain extent, just plain luck.

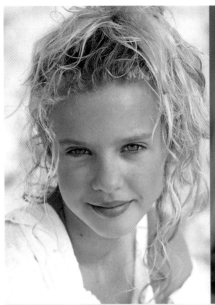 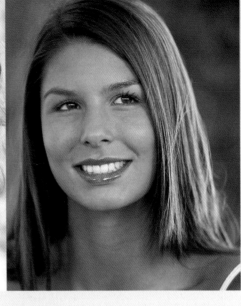

PRE-TEEN

For the first decade of a child's life, its skin looks clear, smooth, plump, wrinkle- and blemish-free. The reason for this healthy appearance is that the epidermis works efficiently – it is translucent and well hydrated. The surface is smooth and unlined and light is reflected from a healthy, undamaged skin, hence the term the 'bloom of youth'. At this age, there is usually little or no apparent sun damage, but it is the time when the damage that will surface later is being done. Now is the time to instil sun awareness in your children. They will thank you 20 years down the line.

TEEN–EARLY 20s

Hormonal changes can cause havoc with skin. They cause an increase in sebum production, which often leads to breakouts, acne and shiny, oily skin. The twenties are a kind of transitional period – by the time you enter them, the extreme hormone production has usually calmed down and your skin becomes normal (although some people suffer from spots well into their 30s). This is the time to establish a good skincare routine. Although the effects of the sun have not become visible, much of the harm will have already been done by the age of 18.

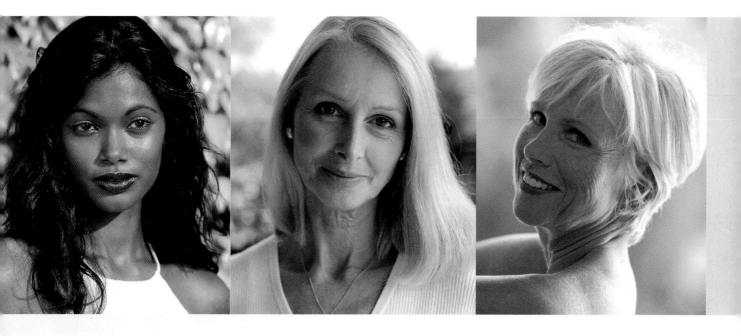

25–40

Towards the end of the twenties, the first signs of fine lines around the eyes and mouth usually appear as collagen and elastin start to break down in the skin. There's a significant drop in skin hydration, and adult acne may also occur. Broken veins may appear as tiny red dots on the skin, and brown pigmentation marks and age spots can begin to show. Pores can enlarge and skin may become coarser due to sun damage, or the fact that the rate of loss of dead surface cells has started to slow down (which is why exfoliation is so important now).

INTO MENOPAUSE

If you looked after yourself in your younger years, you will see the benefits now. At this age natural ageing becomes more visible and deeper wrinkles, crow's feet and frown lines become prominent. Skin loses its firmness as there is a significant decrease in dermal repair and cohesion between the skin's layers. During menopause, the production of oestrogen drops dramatically, causing a breakdown in collagen, resulting in wrinkles and sagging. Skin also becomes more fragile and you may experience slow-healing cuts or bruises.

55+

With decreased thickness of the dermis, decreased resilience of the skin and the loss of subcutaneous fat, sagging and jowl-like wrinkles become apparent. You may also notice an increase in fine facial hair. Skin can appear sallow with uneven colour and dark under-eye circles. If you were a sun worshipper in the past, discolouration will now become visible. You'll notice the effects of gravity most strongly in your 70s – facial skin and neck start to appear 'loose'. Hands, too, will show the passing of time and age spots are pronounced.

The keys to healthy skin

There is no denying the benefits of exercise – it's the easiest way to perk up a lacklustre complexion.

▼

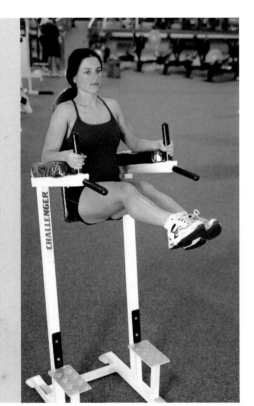

GOOD GENES

You can choose your friends, but not your family – or your genes. Genes play an important part in your overall appearance and determine how your skin behaves and ages. Although you cannot do anything about the characteristics you inherit from your parents, you can use them as an 'age barometer' and take certain steps to arm yourself against problems that are likely to come your way.

REGULAR EXERCISE

During exercise the circulation is boosted and oxygen-rich blood is delivered to every cell in your body allowing nutrients to be absorbed quicker. The short-term effect is a glowing complexion. Long-term, many experts believe that exercise improves the skin's elasticity and encourages new cell growth. Remember, however, that moderation is the key to good health. Professional sportspeople sometimes have a gaunt look due to a low body fat concentration. That is not necessarily a good thing as you get older, as it may mean you lose some of that youthful plumpness. Training outdoors also potentially means more sun exposure.

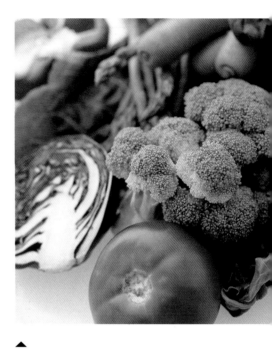

▲

Raw fruit and vegetables are one of the best sources of antioxidant vitamins, vital for good skin.

BALANCED DIET

Although some dermatologists don't believe that what you eat has any effect on the state of your skin, it is acknowledged that your skin reflects the general health of your body. Clear, radiant skin is dependant on the efficient functioning of your kidneys, intestines and liver – the organs responsible for detoxification and waste removal. Excess alcohol, drugs and fatty foods can put strain on these organs, resulting in a sluggish system and pasty, blotchy skin, while smoking and high caffeine intake can compromise your body's defence system. Regular crash dieting also plays havoc with your body and can add as much as 10 years to your face, while nutrient deficiencies will affect your complexion. A lack of protein, for example, can manifest in a dull, dry complexion; a shortage of vitamin C may result in dullness and easy bruising; lack of vitamin A can cause dry skin and a disruption in cellular turnover; a deficiency in iron can produce a pale complexion; and a vitamin B deficiency may lead to breakouts, pallor and cracks at the corners of the mouth.

ENOUGH SLEEP

Skincare experts now believe that skin cells regenerate as the body rests, repairing damage done during the day and producing new cells in preparation for the next. Studies have also shown that sleep-deprived people have lower levels of a growth hormone that influences specific skin-growth factors like collagen and keratin production. As far as most of us are concerned, there's just no denying what a lack of sleep does to your eyes and complexion!

DEEP BREATHING

Your skin absorbs a small amount of oxygen through the pores and so needs to 'breathe'. Try not putting anything onto your face for at least a small part of each day and always cleanse well to avoid blocked pores. Breathing properly through your lungs will also benefit your skin: breathing in supplies your skin with oxygen and breathing out removes carbon dioxide and waste. Many of us breathe incorrectly by taking shallow breaths into the top of the chest.

▼

Try inhaling and exhaling slowly through the nose. Keep the shoulders relaxed and draw each breath right down into your stomach, holding it there to a count of four, before exhaling slowly, emptying out your lungs completely. Breathing is a great stress reliever: it has been shown to lower the pulse rate and its easy, rhythmic quality is comforting.

Sleep allows your body to regenerate and your mind to clear so that you wake up feeling and looking fresh.

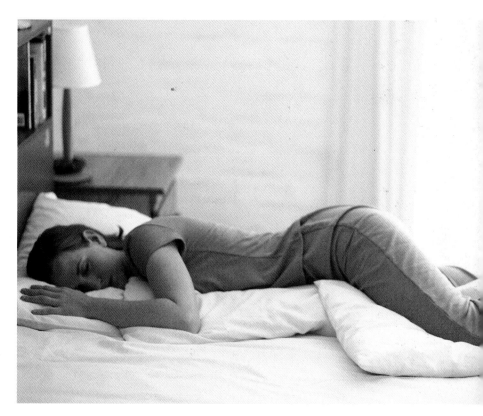

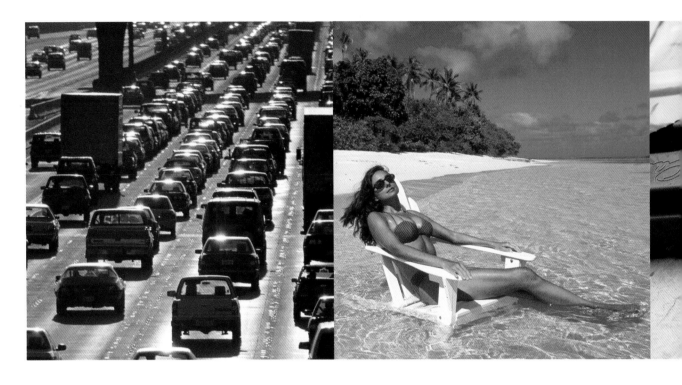

Enemies of the skin

CITY LIFE

Fresh air combined with certain health keys is what we should all aspire to. Unfortunately, modern lifestyles mean it's impossible to escape the city's by-products. There's no doubt that living in a city contributes to premature age-ing of the skin. Chemicals such as car-bon monoxide, oxides of nitrogen, lead and chlorofluorocarbons (all part of what we know as pollution) set off free radicals, which lead to collagen and elastin breakdown. Furthermore, car fumes (especially leaded petrol) and dust can filter in through air vents; chemicals are released into the air by machines; modern ventilation systems restrict the supply of fresh air in office buildings; and there's UV radiation from unnatural light sources and computer screens. Our drinking water often contains chemicals, residues of heavy metals and human wastes. Add stress to this package and it's no wonder we're seeing so many more cases of sensitized skin. In fact, living in a polluted city can add as much as five years to your face. The answer – other than retiring to the Alps – comes in the form of antioxi-dants, which are discussed in depth in chapter two (see p36).

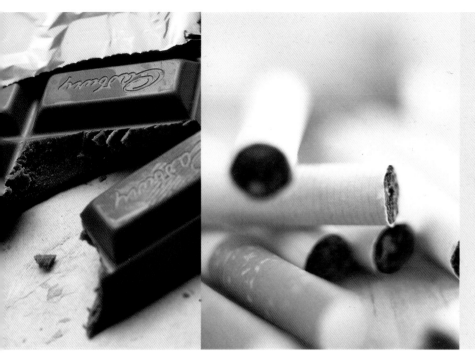

Pollution, sun exposure, sugar and cigarette smoke all trigger the formation of free radicals. The result is a skin 'breakdown' manifesting in premature ageing or even severe conditions such as skin cancer.

SUN

Let's face it, there is no such thing as a healthy tan. While a teeny bit of sun exposure is necessary for vitamin D production, too much sun will prematurely age the skin (see chapter three). According to dermatologists, the sun's ultraviolet rays are accountable for more skin damage than any other factor.

SUGAR

A diet too high in sugar or simple carbohydrates may have a negative effect on the skin's appearance and how fast it ages. Sugar in the human body can attach itself to structural proteins like elastin and collagen, causing them to be less flexible and potentially more prone to degeneration. If, for instance, an enzyme that repairs skin after sun exposure isn't working properly because it's got a sugar stuck to it, then that important function isn't going to happen. Remember that the body converts anything that's starch – rice, pasta, cake and flour – into sugar. Rather opt for 'good' foods like protein, essential fatty acids (found in fatty fish like mackerel, salmon and tuna) and iron. An iron deficiency contributes to anaemia and a low blood count, and produces a pale, sallow complexion.

SMOKING

If you cannot give up smoking for all the sound health reasons, at least consider what it does to your face. The skin of a smoker is, on average, 40% thinner than a non-smoker's. Smokers have far more wrinkles than non-smokers – in fact, a 40-year-old smoker is likely to have as many as a 60-year-old non-smoker. Particularly noticeable are the lines around the mouth (from puckering) and eyes (from squinting through the smoke).

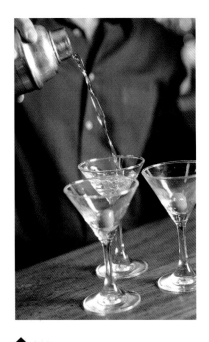

Remember to be moderate in your consumption of alcohol. A glass of wine per day is perfectly permissible, but don't be tempted to overdo it – your skin will pay the price.

Skin, the body's largest organ, makes up about 15% of your body weight.

Furthermore, nicotine and tar slow down the blood circulation and thus reduce blood flow to the skin, depriving it of vital nutrients and oxygen, and leading to an unattractive grey-tinged, dull complexion. The two harmful substances also promote the formation of free radicals and weaken the collagen and elastin fibres, resulting in skin that is prematurely wrinkled. If that's not enough to put you off, consider that smokers have much higher rates of skin cancers, they are less able to utilize antioxidant vitamins such as vitamin C and their wounds heal slower. When your skin is cut, it needs more oxygen and nutrients than normal for the healing process. Smoking causes the little blood vessels in the skin to constrict, resulting in less blood flowing to the skin and therefore slower healing.

ALCOHOL

Alcohol is a toxin and when ingested has to be detoxified by the body. Excessive quantities are not easily dealt with as they place strain on the organs involved in the detoxifying process, such as the liver. While a glass of wine with your meal is fine, a single night of bingeing will be visible on your skin the next morning

as dehydration, redness and puffy eyes. Usually heavy drinkers tend to have heavier capillary formation, giving the skin a red, ruddy look. Alcohol is also a vasodilator: when you drink, your skin feels warm because your blood vessels actually relax, allowing more blood flow to the skin. If you do this consistently, the blood vessels eventually start to stretch, which leads to greater blood vessel formation. Alcohol also depletes the body's levels of vitamin B, especially folic acid and thiamine. In your skin, a deficiency will manifest as a sallow complexion, dryness, slackness and breakouts.

STRESS

Mental overload and undue stress can cause your skin to behave badly. When you're stressed, the body releases adrenal or stress hormones, which bring about a number of changes in the skin, including blemishes and oily or dry patches. In chronic cases, blood is pumped away from the skin to the main organs, resulting in a pale, ashen appearance and under-eye circles. At the same time, cell turnover is slowed, and this leads to a build-up of toxins that makes the skin look sallow.

What are free radicals?

Free radicals are reactive molecules created naturally by the body, particularly when it is exposed to sunlight or under stress. Excessive exercise can also trigger abnormal free radical production due to the increased intake of oxygen. The smoke, chemicals and toxins that we encounter in everyday city life cause almost continual free radical production (the skin can generate free radicals in a millionth of a second if exposed to cigarette smoke).

Free radicals are unstable molecules that act as scavengers in the skin, damaging connective tissue, cell membranes and DNA, our basic genetic building blocks. On the skin, this chemical chaos results in a heightened skin cancer risk and premature ageing. Young, healthy skin has sufficient enzymes and vitamins to neutralize these 'terrorists', but as we age, our natural defense mechanisms become depleted and the skin becomes less effective at defending itself from attack. Antioxidants are currently our best method of limiting free radical damage. They work by stopping the formation of free radicals and 'mopping them up' as they form.

How do free radicals form?

- Oxygen molecules have four pairs of electrons. Sun, smoking, stress, etc. can cause the loss of electrons. At this stage the molecule, desperate to 'regain' its lost electron, is defined as a free radical. So begins the raid on other molecules.

- Scavenging free radicals take an electron from other molecules, thus creating new free radicals that go on their own rampage.

- This chain reaction eventually causes the cell membrane to disintegrate, leaving the cell vulnerable to premature ageing and disease.

- Antioxidants remove free radicals as they form by replacing the lost electrons and so creating normal oxygen molecules.

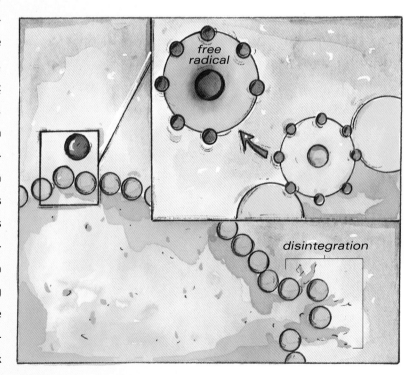

free radical

disintegration

Taking care of your face

Achieving perfect skin many seem impossible to most of us, but we are all capable of having and maintaining good skin. This simply requires getting to know our skin and looking after it – and it's never too early to start. Looking after your skin may mean different things to different people. To some it means washing their face with soap and water and slapping on sun block at the beach; to others it's a regular cleanse and moisturize routine. To many it means spending loads of cash on all the latest wrinkle-reducing, complexion-clearing, blemish-busting lotions and potions. But good skincare doesn't have to be expensive, time consuming or daunting. Before bothering to spend a fortune on products that may not suit you, you need to know your skin type. If you're unsure, go to a professional dermatologist, skincare therapist or beauty advisor at a cosmetics counter for a skin analysis. Your skin is a living organ and can change from season to season – or week to week – depending on your general health, lifestyle, diet and hormonal changes, as well as external factors such as the weather. It is therefore important to have your skin profiled at least twice a year.

Invest in a nourishing moisturizer and eye cream. You can save money on your cleanser and toner.

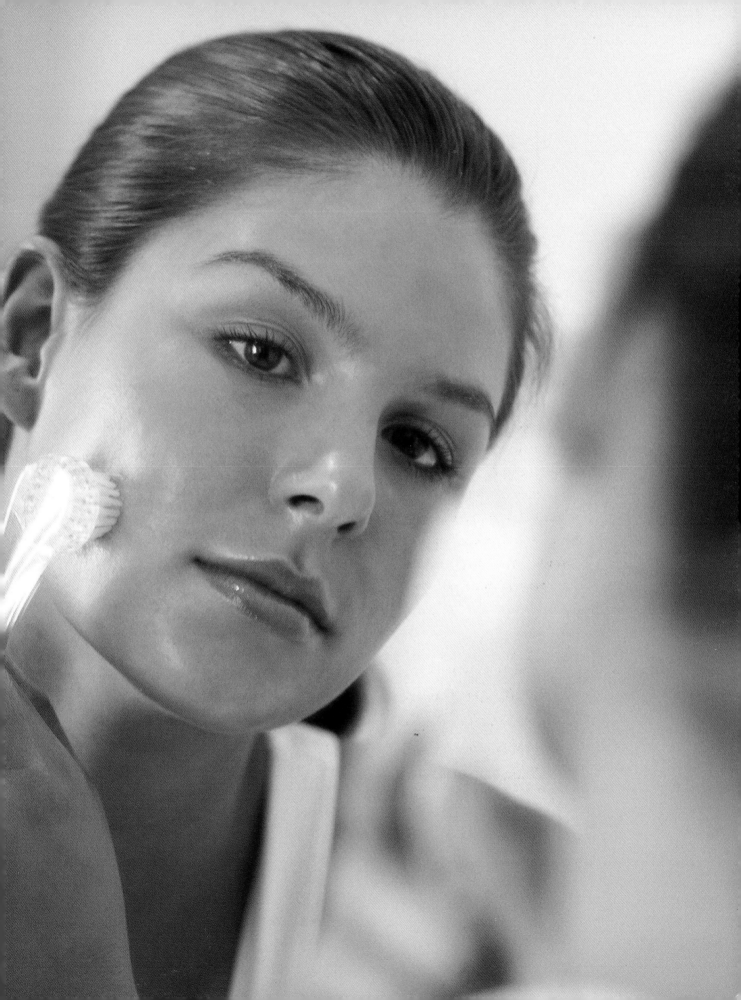

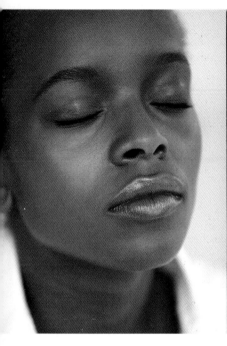
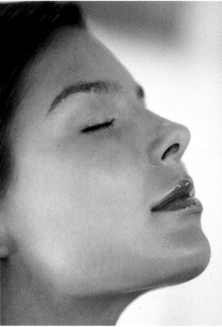
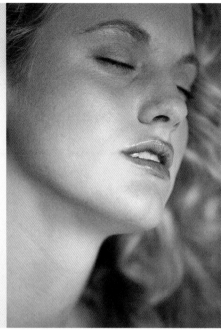

Skin types

Skin types are as individual as personalities, but there are some generally accepted principles. Scientific definitions of skin types are determined by how the skin responds to sun exposure, its ability to tan and hair colour. A very fair person that always burns in the sun would be categorized as a skin type one, while a black-skinned person who rarely burns and tans darkly would be a skin type six. When buying skincare products however, it's often more practical to choose according to how dry or oily your skin feels.

NORMAL SKIN

Normal skin has nothing obviously wrong with it. It is in a balanced state of suppleness, elasticity, hydration and colour, and feels soft and smooth to the touch. It rarely breaks out and feels comfortable after cleansing (neither tight nor dry). Normal skin can change however, as a poor skincare routine, excessive sun, wind or cold exposure, a poor diet and hormones can take their toll.

DRY SKIN

Dry skin is often characterized by feelings of tightness due to a lack of emollients or oil. It has a fine texture, no

You need to know your skin type and identify your key concerns before you put anything on your face.

visible pores, may be rough and scaly in places and shows lines and wrinkles easily. It rarely suffers breakouts. The problem lies in poor epidermal function and damage to the water / lipid barrier. This is a common complaint with mature skin as hydration ability decreases as we age (due to a slowing down of oil production by the sebaceous glands). As the levels of natural lipids and oils drop, the skin's ability to retain water is also reduced, leaving the skin dry and often dehydrated. In young people, a dry skin is usually a result of low sebum production, or it may be that the skin has temporarily dried out as a result of sunburn, extremes of climate, detergents or air conditioning. Dehydrated skin should not be confused with dry skin, although it can feel tight and flaky. Deeply nourishing or hydrating masks and moisturizers can be used to rebalance the skin and help to prevent against further moisture loss.

OILY SKIN

Greasy or oily skin is particularly common in teenagers and young adults, but much less so after the age of 35. A result of excess sebum production, it's characterized by a shiny appearance, especially on the 'T-zone' – the forehead, nose and chin. The epidermis tends to thicken and the pores dilate, giving the skin a slightly rough and irregular texture. A person with this skin type is more likely to suffer from spots and acne.

COMBINATION SKIN

There are two forms of combination skin: oily/normal and dry/normal. In oily/normal combination skin, the

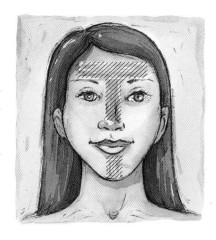

▲

This illustration depicts the location of the T-zone – an oily area that's prone to breakouts, and usually develops a shine during the day.

centre panel (T-zone) is oily while the rest of the face is comfortable. In the dry/normal combination skin, the centre panel may be normal with dry patches on the cheeks. You need to treat both zones in combination skin – moisturizing the dry patches and controlling the sebum on the oily parts.

SENSITIVE VERSUS SENSITIZED?

In addition to these skin types, many people believe they have sensitive skin. However, true sensitivity is not as common as we think. Truly sensitive skin is easily irritated and cannot

tolerate cosmetic products. Many of us suffer bouts of skin sensitivity, set off by anything from climate changes to stress. This is a temporary state, referred to as sensitized skin, and can usually be relieved through soothing treatment. The best way to handle sensitive skin is by treating it as though it's very dry: don't scrub or exfoliate, have facials nor use masks unless you are certain that the products suit you. Steer clear of soap, which can alter the skin's natural pH balance, alpha hydroxy creams, the sun and perfumes. Look for hypoallergenic and allergy tested products or consult a dermatologist. A sensitive skin is slightly different to an allergic skin. While sensitivity is difficult to cure, with the right products it can be significantly improved. Allergic skin, on the other hand, tends to react more aggressively and the reaction may last for up to 10 days. These skin types may need a dermatological skincare routine. If your skin is behaving badly, it may be a sign that your body is taking strain – in times of stress, your skin gets the short end of the stick. The bottom line: take a look at your lifestyle and see how you can reduce stress in order to gain control of your skin.

Basics of skincare

CLEANSE

Cleansing is one of the single most important things you can do for your skin. Everyone's skin gets dirty from dust, sweat, make-up, sebum and impurities in the air. If you do not cleanse, your pores will become clogged and your skin will start to look dull. Choosing a cleanser has a lot to do with personal preference, but always take your skin type into account. Cream cleansers are rich and gentle and leave a light, moisturizing film on the skin, which is ideal for dry, sensitive and mature skins. The drier your skin, the richer the cleanser you'll need. A lotion or gel cleanser is ideal for normal skin as it rinses off easily, while foaming cleansers are best used on greasy skin as they dissolve any excess oil on the skin. Avoid scrubbing acne-prone skin as it may irritate the lesions. Soap is a no-no on your face. Your skin is by nature slightly acidic (with a pH of about 5.5) and most soap leaves an alkaline residue that's difficult to wash off and may leave skin feeling dry and tight. If you just can't wean yourself off that lathering texture, some cosmetics houses make soap-free 'facial bars' that foam, but are gentler than regular soap. Generally, if you have very dry skin, it's advisable to avoid soap bars altogether.

How often should I cleanse?

Cleansing twice a day is sufficient. If you are using mild and well-formulated products you won't damage the skin. Some experts believe you should have at least two cleansers – a milder formula for the morning when there's little or no oil build-up, and a deeper cleansing product for the end of the day.

TONE

The jury is still out on toners. Many dermatologists believe that they don't provide any special benefit other than to remove the final traces of make-up and cleanser and so make the skin feel clean and fresh. They cannot actually 'close' pores as some manufacturers claim they do – pores are the openings for the sebaceous glands and can't be closed from the outside. However, modern formulations are becoming more and more sophisticated, with some offering soothing and anti-ageing benefits.

It is true that certain exfoliating or clarifying lotions can make your skin look more radiant by dissolving dead surface cells. Many brands also claim that toners help to restore the pH balance of the skin after cleansing. Astringents are strong toners with a high alcohol content that may irritate some sensitive and dry skins. Many toners that are designed for use on oily skins contain alcohol precisely because of its drying effect. However, they can also aggravate acne-prone skin as they may cause an increase in the skin's oil production as well as increased sensitivity.

MOISTURIZE

In the past, moisturizers were designed simply to serve as barriers against the environment. Neither did they penetrate the skin, nor allow it to 'breathe', thus leading to congested, nutrient-starved skin.

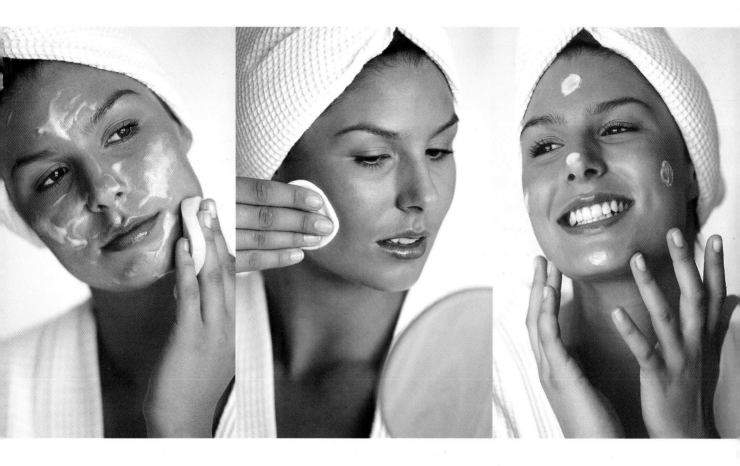

Modern moisturizers are designed to help the skin function properly and to improve water retention in the epidermis by 'sealing' it – effectively maintaining a delicate balance between adding water to the surface and preventing evaporation. A vast choice of products is available and it is hard to decide which moisturizer is right for you. As a guideline, we should all be wearing a moisturizer that offers antioxidant benefits (to fight free radicals and prevent premature ageing). The majority of modern formulations also contain a myriad other ingredients to firm, smooth, mattify or boost radiance, for example. Ask yourself what concerns you most about your skin – is it your breakouts, pigmentation, fine lines, dryness, lack of radiance or wrinkles? – and choose accordingly. As a general rule, drier skins needs a rich, hydrating moisturizer, while combination and oily skins do better with a lightweight lotion. If your moisturizer does not contain a sunscreen, layer one over it.

▲

Cleansing your skin not only improves the way you look, properly cleansed skin will be more receptive to active ingredients in your treatment products, so they will work better.

benefits. If your skin suffers from excessive dryness during winter, for example, a hydrating serum can be used just for those few months until the weather changes and your skin is back to normal.

Eye cream

Because the skin around the eyes is the first to show signs of ageing, there is definitely a case for using a special cream for this area. The skin around the eyes ages more quickly because it is thinner than that on the rest of the face, and so is less able to retain moisture. Also, the area is generally more sensitive, with fewer and smaller oil glands and, because the eyes are so expressive, the skin around them is made to move excessively. If you use your regular moisturizer around the eye area you could end up with puffy, irritated eyes, while rich lotions can block the glands.

The fragrances, emulsifiers and emollients that are used in various moisturizers and night creams may also cause sensitivity in this delicate area. Most eye products have multiple benefits, targeting the common problems associated with the skin around the eyes like fine lines, dark circles and puffiness.

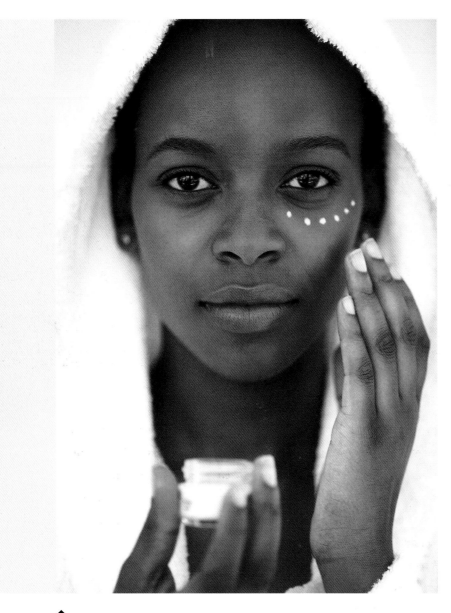

▲

Never apply eye cream directly to the eyelid or underneath the eye. Using your ring finger, dot it on the orbital bone that circles the eye. The product will gradually work its way in through the repeated action of blinking.

Serums and boosters

These lightweight formulations have a high concentration of active ingredients and are ideal for special care. Applied under your moisturizer, they usually have anti-ageing or hydrating

Neck cream

Because the skin on the neck has a small number of fat cells and low supplies of sebum, it is prone to dryness and sagging and, like your hands, reveals your age. A specially enriched neck cream, therefore, has its benefits, but you can also just extend your regular routine to the décolletage.

Do I really need a serum, night cream, eye gel, and neck cream?

In addition to moisturizers, there's a whole host of potions out there that you've probably been told are essential to a good skincare routine. Many dermatologists scoff at them; many skincare experts swear by their added benefits. While there's only so much your skin can absorb, how many extras you want to add to your basic routine is up to you. If in doubt, consult a professional.

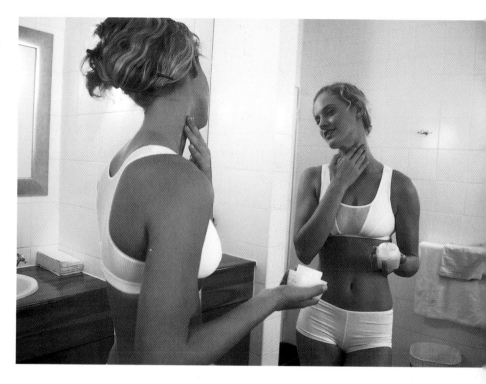

Night cream

According to our internal clocks, different body cells are more active at certain times of the day. Skin cells do their repair work most effectively at night. In fact, research shows that skin cell regeneration almost doubles at night, peaking between 23:00 and 4:00. Production of collagen (the skin's natural support structure) is boosted, harmful free radicals are destroyed and cell damage is rectified. The latest night creams are designed to maximize the nighttime repair process and are generally more nourishing than a day cream.

▲

The neck and décolletage are often exposed, so protect and treat them with the same care as you do your face by simply extending your skincare routine down to your chest.

31

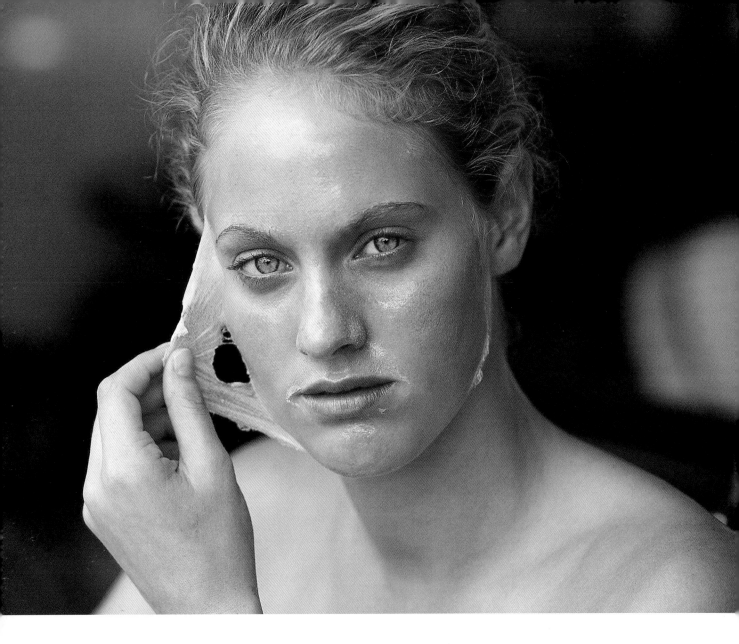

▲

Whether you want to smooth, purify, hydrate, brighten or soothe your skin, there's a face mask for you. Masks should be used regularly for the best results, but do not overuse them.

MASKS

Applied to cleansed skin, a good mask can be an instant beauty fix. Masks are generally fairly concentrated and infuse skin with beneficial ingredients. There are various types of masks to choose from. As a guide, clay, mud or peel-off masks are best for deep cleansing and perfect for oily skin, while dry skin will benefit from a rich,

hydrating treatment. Masks that claim to replenish, perfect or boost radiance are ideal to pep up a dull complexion. Masks and serums are also the perfect way to treat temporary skin conditions such as dehydration or some form of sensitivity, caused by environmental factors. They can be applied once or twice a week depending on the severity of your problem.

Exfoliate to rejuvenate

Our largest organ of elimination, the skin sheds around five billion dead cells daily. One of the reasons young skin is so clear and radiant is because in its prime, young, healthy skin replaces itself naturally every 14 days. As age sets in this process slows until, at about age 40, the renewal cycle is increased to 30 days. If these dead skin cells sit on the surface of the skin, they clog the pores and make the complexion look dull. Removing them reveals clearer, brighter skin and restores suppleness and vigour by stimulating cell renewal.

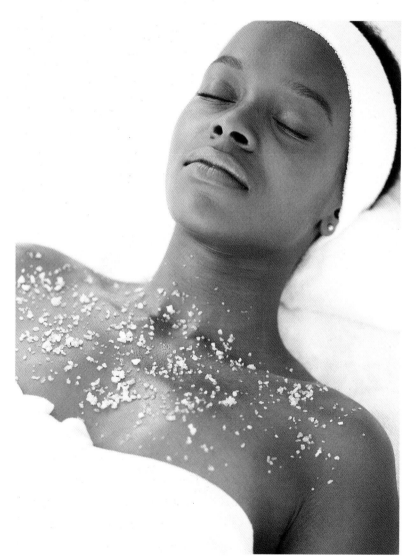

Myth: Use a deep-cleansing grainy scrub to open clogged pores and remove dead skin over a breakout.

Fact: Use a gentle, nonabrasive exfoliant to smooth the skin's surface and prevent further breakouts, unless you're on Roaccutane or Retin-A; these products already provide a peeling action.

◀

Exfoliating too often or too harshly can compromise your skin's protective waterproof layer. Be very careful of abrasive products; ideally thorough exfoliations should be done by a skincare therapist.

33

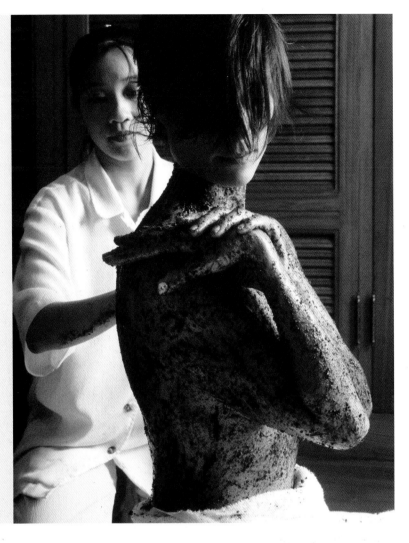

Your entire body will benefit from a thorough exfoliation procedure. It is particularly useful before applying a self-tanning lotion, as the product is much less likely to leave unsightly streaks when applied to smooth skin.

Many of the newer scrubs contain tiny encapsulated beads to ensure a gentle exfoliation process that does not abrade unnecessarily.

Alpha hydroxy acids (fruit acids) are a group of natural chemicals found in fruit, wine, sugar cane and sour milk that exfoliate the skin's surface layer and accelerate new cell production. If you use products that contain these ingredients on a daily basis, avoid combining them with abrasive scrubs. Always be very gentle as over-exfoliation can cause sensitivity. By removing too many cells you could compromise the skin's natural protective barrier and reveal cells that have not been properly primed for the harsh environment.

There are various ways to exfoliate:

- **Mechanical exfoliation** involves products like synthetic buffing beads, scrubs containing apricot kernels, a muslin face cloth or facial brush. If you like to use a scrub, look for a gentle one with fine granules that dissolve in water. Don't overdo it – once a week is enough.

- **Chemical exfoliants** have ingredients like alpha and beta hydroxy acids, retinoic acid or enzymes (such as papain, found in papaya). These literally 'unglue' dead surface cells and do not require vigorous rubbing and rinsing.

Organic versus natural

There is a definite shift towards harnessing the healing power of nature, and the production and consumption of organic and 'natural' skincare products is increasing. The question is: how natural is 'natural' and what exactly is the difference between natural and organic? If a product is truly organic it will be certified by an organic certification agency. The trouble is that it's hard to produce 100% organic beauty products because preservatives are vital constituents, and natural preservatives are hard to find.

Natural products are made from plants and minerals that occur in nature and have not been produced in a laboratory. Organic products are also made from natural ingredients; they are grown without the use of chemicals or pesticides. Seaweed, for example, can be classified as a natural product, but is not organic because it's not grown in controlled conditions.

Truly organic products do not contain any genetically modified ingredients nor petrochemicals (synthetic ingredients derived from natural petroleum or oil), nor do they undergo any animal testing (unless required by law) and are only subjected to minimal processing. Some cosmetic companies add natural ingredients in the form of fruit acids, vitamins, borage and hemp to skincare products. Some products use ingredients that mimic the skin's natural functions, like hyaluronic acid, a moisturizer that occurs naturally in the skin.

So what is best? Some experts believe that 60% of everything you put on your skin is absorbed by it. Your skin is a highly effective delivery system, so it makes sense that organic beauty products – made without the use of artificial fertilizers, pesticides, chemicals or drugs – ensure the highest level of nourishment to the skin. But remember that you can still have an allergic reaction to a 'natural' product. Natural ingredients can trigger skin reactions in the same way that synthetic ingredients can. If you have sensitive skin, look for products that have full ingredient listings to enable you to identify potential aggressors. (See p36 for more information.)

▲

Seaweed has detoxifying properties – it stimulates circulation and encourages the elimination of wastes and water.

35

A SKIN FOR ALL SEASONS

Winter can be torture to your skin, so it's no surprise that many recurrent skin problems are at their worst at this time of year. Dryness can diminish the epidermis' ability to provide protection, leading to seasonal eczema, hypersensitivity and rough skin. With a little care, however, you can keep your skin looking its best come rain or shine. During dry weather, the key is more moisture, more often. If you use an oil-free moisturizer, consider upgrading to one that contains small amounts of essential oils for a moisture boost, or switch from your summer moisturizer to a richer cream. Depending on the humidity levels, you may also want to apply a weekly hydrating mask to help restore suppleness to the skin. Putting a humidifier in your home and office will also help prevent dehydration, which is especially important if you are constantly exposed to air-conditioners and heaters.

INGREDIENT WATCH

Alpha hydroxy acids (AHAs) or fruit acids, are derived from natural ingredients such as milk, olives, apples and grapes. They help speed up the exfoliation process by dissolving the glue that bonds the cells. When choosing an AHA, it's important to consider the form and concentration. Lactic acid (made from fermented milk) and glycolic acid (made from sugar cane), for example, are particularly effective in treating dry skin and dry-skin diseases such as eczema and psoriasis, as well as decreasing wrinkles. Regarding the concentration: the higher it is, the more effective is the product. However, AHAs should be used with caution. They can cause irritation and do increase the skin's sensitivity to the sun. If you use AHAs, you need to use a daily sunscreen with SPF15 or higher.

Antioxidants are part of the body's natural defence system, derived from vitamins A, C and E. They protect the skin by attaching themselves to free radicals and neutralizing them. Since your skin is your first line of defence against the outside world it makes sense to arm it with the most potent antioxidants available. Other good antioxidants include grape seed extract, black and green tea extract and lycopene (extracted from tomatoes, red guava, watermelon and the skin of red grapes). Polyphenols or

Did you know? Vitamin C applied topically to the skin protects it against free radicals for two to three days. And, since it does not wash off, it delivers extra long-lasting benefits.

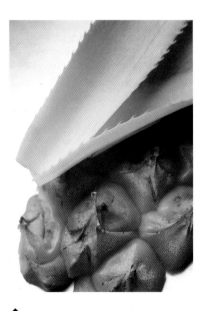
▲

Fruit or vegetable pulp can make a wonderful skin treatment. It contains stimulating enzymes that can make the skin look firmer and fresher.

catechins, which are found in green tea, exhibit powerful antioxidant properties. In fact, they are 20 times stronger than vitamin E.

Beta hydroxy acids (BHAs) work in much the same way as AHAs. The best known of the BHAs is salicylic acid, which is made from willow bark. BHAs appear to be less irritating than AHAs.

Coenzyme Q10 occurs naturally in every skin cell and helps convert food into energy. Without Co-Q10 – known as the 'fuel of youth' – the body's cells are unable to produce energy. Stress, UV radiation and ageing cause a drop in the natural levels of this coenzyme, while increased levels boost cell activity, regeneration and elasticity.

Enzymes like papain (from papaya) and bromelian (from pineapple) are botanically derived and naturally exfoliate and brighten the skin. Enzyme activators are also being designed to suppress the 'bad' enzymes – collagenase and elastase – that damage collagen and elastin.

Flavonoids belong to a group of organic plant molecules produced by plants to protect themselves from attack by diseases and insects as well as damage from intense UV light. Green tea is rich in flavonoid antioxidants. They're also found in onions, apples and citrus fruits. They mop up free radicals, fight off viruses, calm inflammation and help protect against allergies.

Retinoids is a derivative term for vitamin A. Powerful retinoids like retinoic acid are found in prescription-only products like Retin-A and Roaccutane and are used to treat sun damage and acne. Gentler derivatives like retinyl palmitate and retinol can be found in cosmetic creams.

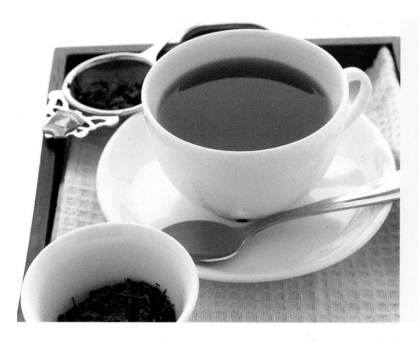

▲

Herb teas are excellent for health and beauty. Green tea, especially, is a superb source of antioxidants.

Vitamins for the skin

Nutrition seems to play an enormous role in minimizing free radical damage. Studies show that after the age of 30, there is a sharp decrease in the number of ingested vitamins that are transported to the skin – and this is when our skin most needs antioxidant protection. However, applying potent, stabilized vitamins to the skin via creams and lotions can significantly help reduce the effects of premature ageing.

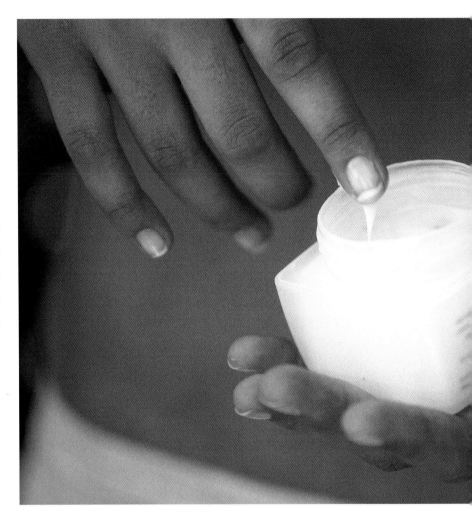

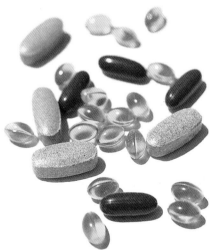

◀

Our hectic, modern lifestyle taxes the body and depletes its natural supply of vitamins and minerals. Adding good vitamin and mineral supplements to your diet can boost your immune system and improve the way you look and feel.

▲

Eating a diet rich in antioxidant vitamins and using an antioxidant cream on a daily basis is a wise insurance policy for your skin. Look out for products that contain vitamin A (to act on wrinkles), vitamin C (for radiance and tone) and vitamin E (to improve texture).

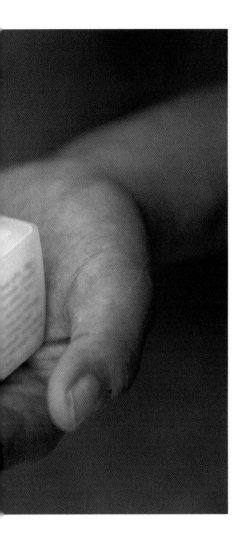

THE BENEFITS OF TOPICALLY APPLIED VITAMINS

Vitamin A

- Improves skin elasticity
- Increases moisture content, making skin appear more supple
- Helps to reverse the signs of photo ageing
- Scavenges free radicals

Vitamin C

- Plays a vital role in the production of pro collagen, the building blocks of collagen fibres
- Controls production of hyperpigmentation
- Scavenges free radicals
- Strengthens capillary walls; helps heal the skin
- Boosts skin's immune system

Vitamin E

- Protects skin cells and membranes
- Controls production of collagen
- Appears to promote skin healing
- Relieves skin dryness
- Slows collagen degradation
- Anti-inflammatory

Pro-Vitamin B5

- Encourages cell regeneration
- Stimulates the healing process
- Prevents scarring
- Conditions the skin

Vitamin F

- Restores the skin's natural barrier function
- Maintains optimum moisture levels

Topically applied vitamins are very fragile. When exposed to oxygen, light or pollution, they can decompose and lose many of their beneficial qualities. Look for sealed packages that are specifically designed to protect the potency of products, as opposed to vitamin-rich skin-care products that are packaged in open containers such as jars or dropper bottles.

39

Sun savvy

Despite all warnings to the contrary, come summer, the beaches are packed as we bare our bodies to get a tan. While a small amount of early-morning sun is good for you (15 minutes is sufficient to provide you with natural vitamin D, and occasional exposure is believed to improve psychological wellbeing), too much sun is dangerous. Besides the fact that sun dramatically ages your skin, it is also the cause of several kinds of skin cancer, including solar keratoses (wart-like growths) and malignant melanoma – and just one bout of harsh sunburn may be all it takes. Photo ageing – which can make up to around 85% of the overall appearance of ageing – is a slow process and only becomes visible after a few decades. And then it's too late to do anything about it.

Wrinkles and other sun-related signs of premature ageing begin to form up to 10 years before they actually appear.

Unfortunately, although people are now waking up to the dangers of overexposure and the horrors of skin cancer, only about half of the world's population takes adequate precautions to protect themselves from the sun. Sun safety should be a vital part of your life and one that you must instil in your children from an early age.

40

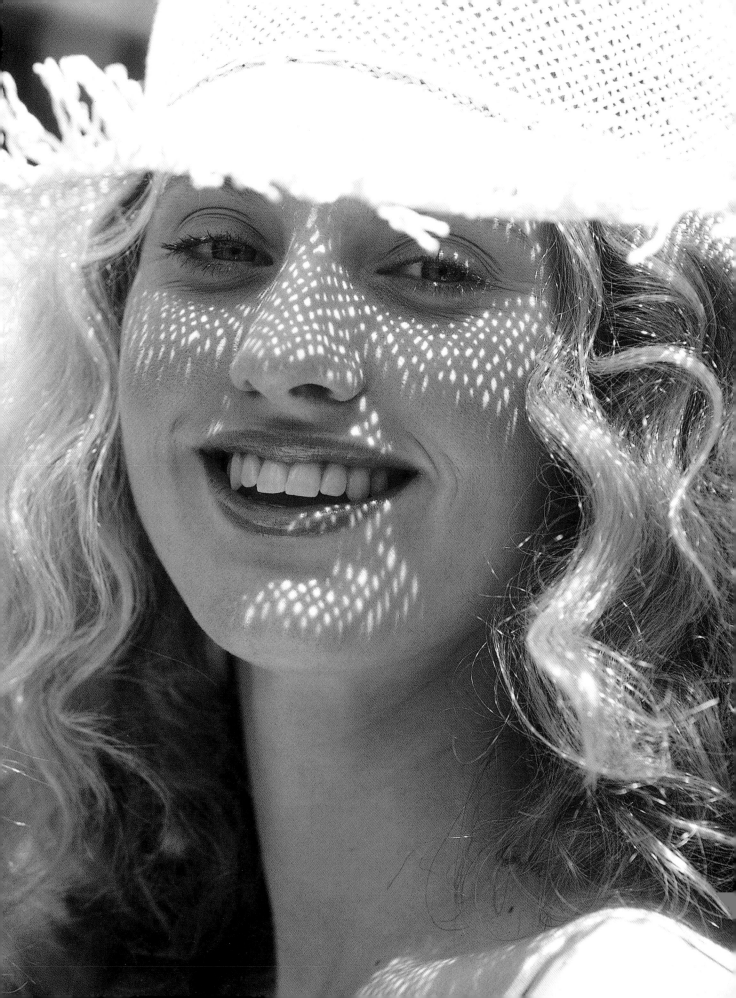

The sun and your skin

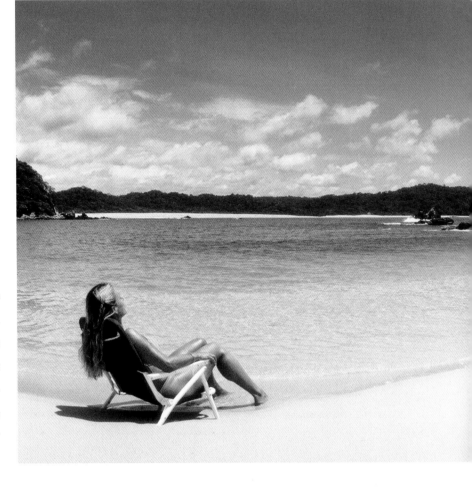

▶

Your best ally against premature ageing is the daily use of a good sunscreen. The higher the SPF (Sun Protection Factor), the oilier the cream generally is. So if you're prone to breakouts stick to SPF 15 or lower or try a gel formula.

Photo ageing, a result of sun exposure, is a slow process. It may take several decades before it becomes fully noticeable. In fact, 90% of sun damage occurs by the age of 20, only becoming visible in your early thirties and onwards. The degree of photo ageing is mainly determined by your skin type and total lifetime sun exposure, and the degree of damage to different areas of the body is directly proportional to the amount of sunlight received (your hands and neckline for example, are more likely to have sun damage and age spots than your stomach). Seriously sun-damaged skin has a thickened outer layer, making it feel dry, rough and leathery. There are often darkly pigmented areas or whitish spots where levels of pigment are higher or lower than normal. Pores may be dilated and small blood vessels become more obvious, sometimes forming broken or spider-like veins, and the skin may be mottled red or inflamed. Within the dermis, the elastic fibres increase in quantity and thickness, manifesting as deep, fixed wrinkles and less pliable skin.

THE SCIENCE OF SUNBURN

The sun energy that reaches the Earth can be divided into three kinds of light: infrared and visible light, and ultraviolet radiation (UVR). UVR, in turn, consists of three different wavelengths: ultraviolet A, B and C.

- **Ultraviolet C** is the shortest wavelength and potentially the most damaging. DNA and proteins absorb UVC due to their molecular structure. Fortunately for us, UVC is mostly absorbed in the atmosphere by the ozone layer. However, the current 'thinning' of this layer has increased the amounts that reach our planet, especially in the Southern Hemisphere.

- **UVB** is the most potent wavelength as it can penetrate into the epidermis where it affects the DNA and can create lipid peroxides, precursors of free radicals. It is believed to generate most of the photo damage to skin. UVB is the wavelength responsible for sunburn, and is at its most dangerous in the middle of a summer day, when transmitted through a blue sky. Less UVB is transmitted in the early mornings and late evenings; when the sun is lowest in the sky.

- **UVA** is about 1 000 times less damaging to the skin than UVB, but it is far from harmless. UVA rays are longer than UVB rays, and 90% of the sunlight reaching the earth is made up of UVA rays. They are the 'ageing' rays, which penetrate deeper into the skin (the dermis) and are responsible for the damage to your collagen and elastin, and causing freckles, blotchiness and pigmentation problems. While UVB peaks at high noon in summer, UVA is fairly constant throughout the day and year and can penetrate cloud cover, tinted glass and clothing relatively easily. UVA also causes immune suppression, resulting in increased susceptibility to skin infections and even skin cancer.

HOW SUNLIGHT PENETRATES THE SKIN

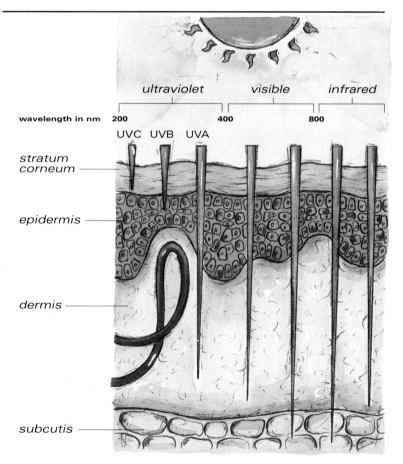

43

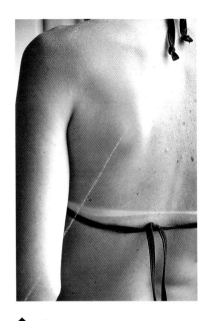

▲

Overexposure to the sun at an early age will result in premature wrinkling between the ages of 25 and 40. The dangerous rays are not just from the sun's light – they are also reflected off water and the earth.

SUNBURN VS SUNTAN

There is no such thing as a safe tan. A suntan is actually the body's defence mechanism against too strong sunlight and the visible evidence of damage to the skin. Sunlight stimulates the skin to increase melanin production. As the melanin supply is activated, it moves up towards the surface of the skin where it helps prevent burning and reduces the penetration of the sun's rays. The side effect is skin of that golden colour that sun worshippers crave. Although dark-skinned people have more melanin in their skin and thus have a higher level of natural protection, they still need to use a sunscreen to avoid skin damage.

Sunburn, on the other hand, can be equated to 'cooking' your skin. If you don't apply sunscreen, or accidentally fall asleep in the sun, the surface blood vessels dilate (hence the redness), and an inflammatory response is induced to fight the damage, often causing blisters in the process. The redness occurs two to eight hours after severe sun exposure and blistering can occur after 12 to 24 hours. A frightening fact is that our skin 'remembers' this burn, and the DNA may not repair perfectly. These 'errors' in DNA can lead to skin

cancer years later. So when you make your way to the coast for your next summer holiday, remember that although a tan fades quickly, your skin carries a permanent memory of the damage.

PROTECTING YOUR SKIN

The time it takes for unprotected skin to turn red in the sun is known as the MED (minimal erythema dose). Your skin type determines your MED. Very fair skin, for example, will have a MED of about six minutes; olive-toned skin can tolerate about 10 to 12 minutes; and black skin usually has a MED of 18 to 20 minutes. SPF (Sun Protection Factor) is a standardized measure that indicates how

Sun-worshipping is the single most destructive activity for your skin, with over 90% of all visible signs of ageing a result of sun exposure.

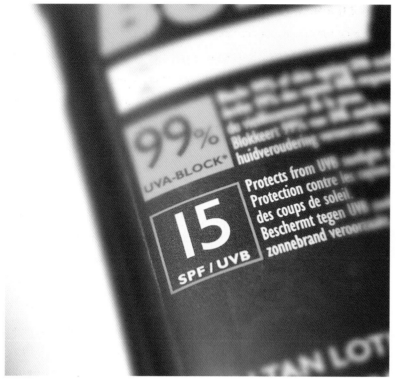

No tanning product can guarantee to tan your skin a certain colour – depth of a tan is determined by the skin's ability to produce melanin. The key to 'safe' tanning is to use a product that allows production of pigment to take place slowly by screening out most of the sun's harmful UV rays.

The rule for choosing a sunscreen: use a moderate filter on your body and high protection for your face.

much additional time above your MED you can spend in the sun without getting burned. For example, if you can usually spend 10 minutes in the sun before burning, an SPF15 sunscreen will multiply that time by fifteen (10 minutes x 15 = 150 minutes of 'sun time'). Note that a person with fair skin can spend far less time in the sun than someone with darker skin, even if they both apply the same level of SPF. Once your time is up, you should ideally get out of the sun. Reapplying sunscreen only means that you will 'cook' more slowly, a bit like cooking your Sunday roast in the oven – once it's done you're simply crisping it! You should, however, always reapply sunscreen after swimming, perspiring and drying yourself off. The key is to use enough sunscreen (one to two ounces) for an even and full coverage. Double application is also important: apply the first layer 20 to 30 minutes before you go to the beach, and apply another layer as your 'coat of armour' when you get into the sun.

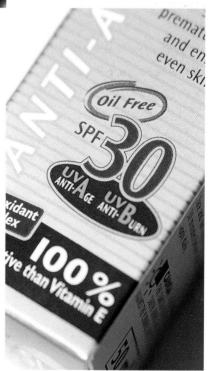

PHYSICAL AND CHEMICAL SUNSCREENS

Sunscreen formulations rely on physical or chemical agents to provide protection. Physical sunscreens contain inert mineral particles that reflect or block UV rays. (Think of the white zinc dioxide layer that the cricketers use.) The molecules cannot break down or be absorbed by the skin and are therefore less likely to irritate the skin. This type of sunscreen is generally better for sensitive skin types. Physical sunscreens of the past tended to be thick, white and greasy, but modern preparations contain ultra-fine titanium dioxide crystals that don't leave that white residue and actually help to absorb oil. Chemical sunscreens, on the other hand, contain synthetic chemical substances that absorb UV radiation. Some of the ingredients can be absorbed through the skin, so these sunscreens may cause irritation. PABA (para-aminobenzoic acid) is one of the most common sensitivity triggers in chemical sunscreens. When choosing a sunscreen, look for ingredients like titanium dioxide or Parsol 1789 (also known as avobenzone; the most effective ingredient for absorbing

Low levels of melanin make light skin much more susceptible to photo ageing. Yet black skin, which has quite a high melanin content, is not immune to sunburn.

▼

Sunburn and sunbeds can add 20 years to your face.

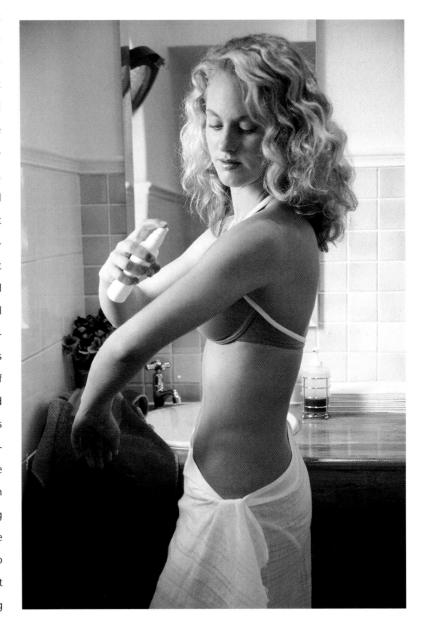

UVA) and do a patch test to check for sensitivity. Make sure any product you choose offers UVA and UVB protection. It's also essential that your sunscreen contains antioxidants such as vitamin E, flavonoids and ascorbic acid to neutralize free radical damage and trigger the repair process. Always choose a product that suits your skin type. For example, gel is best for oily skin, and creams and lotions are most suitable for dry skin.

FAUX GLOWS

What we're hearing from dermatologists is that the only safe tan is one that comes in a tube. The good news is that this is the golden age for bottled tans; the modern formulas can give a natural looking glow without the orange streaks and bad smells of past formulations. Self tans use DHA (dihydroxyacetone), colourless sugar that reacts with dead skin cells to create a tanned effect. The reaction is not immediate; it usually takes three to four hours for the colour to develop fully. As your skin constantly renews itself, fake tans only last five to seven days. It's very important to remember that fake tans do not provide any sun protection, so you still need to wear a sunscreen.

Primary damage is done to your skin while you're in the sun. However, there is a secondary burst of free radical damage for another 24 hours after exposure. To counter this damage, you must get enough antioxidants and make repair part of your skincare routine.

WHAT ABOUT SUNBEDS?

If you are at all concerned about your skin, you should never lie on a sunbed. The ultraviolet light used by indoor tanning systems is as dangerous as that of the sun and although they usually filter out the burning UVB rays, they let the UVA rays in even deeper. Sunbeds are, in essence, automatic ageing machines and increase your risk of melanoma.

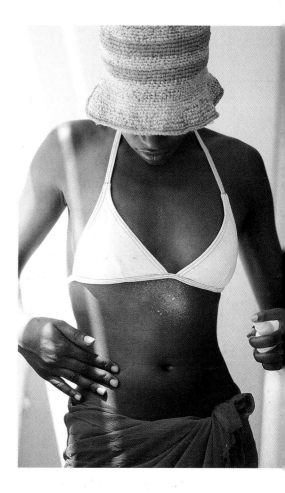

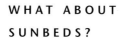

If you do burn in the sun, you can partially alleviate the unpleasant sting by applying cool compresses or adding oatmeal to a lukewarm bath. Creams containing menthol can be very soothing too.

Should I wear a daily sunscreen?

Yes! Eighty percent of all sun exposure is incidental – in other words, walking, driving to work (the side of your face closest to the window will exhibit more signs of premature ageing), or taking a break outdoors. In fact, sitting outside at noon for your lunch hour is worse than being on the beach between 9–11:00 or 14:00–17:00. For this reason, it is generally accepted that everyone should be using some sort of daily sun protection. This is especially important if you are at risk for skin cancer or are on antibiotics, antimalarials, Retin-A, Roaccutane, antidepressants, or some hormone replacement therapies, as they can all increase photosensitivity. So, even when it's overcast, be sure to apply a sunscreen every morning. If you have sensitive skin, rather use a lower SPF and be careful to avoid the sun.

WHY VITAMIN A IS SO VITAL

Vitamin A supports the natural health of the skin. Melanocytes, keratinocytes, fibroblasts and Langerhans cells all depend on vitamin A, and a deficiency will also result in a depletion of vitamin C. Although vitamin A protects the skin from the sun, UVA destroys it. If you spend the weekend tanning next to the swimming pool, for example, the levels of vitamin A in your skin will be depleted and it will take about seven days to restore those levels. Ten minutes in the sun will cause the vitamin A level in the skin to drop to about 40%, while 30 minutes of sun exposure will take the level down to about 10%. To maintain a high enough level of vitamin A in the skin to protect it, it's essential to apply vitamin A topically, and to supply the skin with antioxidants that protect your vitamin stores from attack by free radicals.

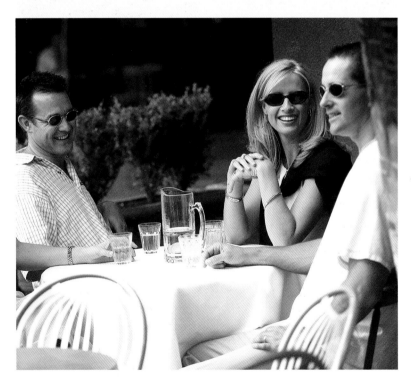

◀

There's no doubt that sunshine makes us feel good. It is essential, however, to learn how to enjoy it without putting your skin at risk.

AND NOW FOR THE GOOD NEWS...

Although for many people the rate of damage is higher than the skin's inherent ability to repair itself, there is a lot of potential for self-repair. The key is to start taking the proper precautions now, if you haven't being doing so already. Always protect yourself from the sun. By simply applying a daily sunscreen, you are giving your skin a chance to 'rest' and conserve some of the energy it would otherwise expend on protection during the day. As these energy reserves grow, your skin has a better chance of carrying out the crucial roles of repairing and rebuilding itself; ensuring long term healthy functioning.

How do I know if I am at risk for skin cancer?

Every person runs some risk of developing skin cancer; a lighter skin tone and unprotected sun exposure increase that risk. It is crucial to protect young skin because a severe burn before the age of 18 almost doubles the risk of skin cancer and premature ageing. After years of sun exposure, basal cell carcinoma and squamous cell carcinoma are the most common types of skin cancer and often appear on exposed areas of the skin. Melanomas are the most widely known type of skin cancer and the deadliest. Remember the ABCD of warning signs for changes in a mole, which may indicate melanoma: **A** is for asymmetry: has its shape changed? **B** is for border: have the edges increased or become irregular? **C** is for colour: has the mole darkened or is the colour not uniform? **D** is for diameter: has it become larger than 6mm (¼in)? Speak to a dermatologist immediately if you answer yes to any of the above questions, or if you are concerned by any suddenly appearing skin lesion. Early detection can make all the difference between successful removal and long-term illness.

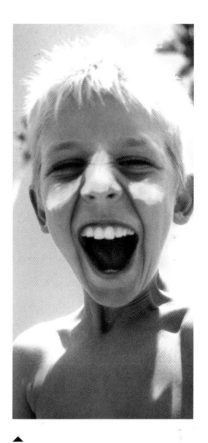

▲

Always remember: how you look after your skin as a child (parents, take note!) will determine your appearance 20 years down the line.

Problem skin

Most of us are born with perfect skin. While a lucky few manage to maintain a clear complexion over the years, most of the rest have experienced a few unwanted changes. For some it may be small irritations such as breakouts, dark patches after a pregnancy or enlarged pores. For others, it may be a more severe skin condition, like eczema or acne. Everyone experiences marks and blemishes on their skin at some point. Some are permanent, others tend to come and go. Most will be of no importance, while some may require a professional opinion. While you can never regain the skin you were born with, there are many things you can do to improve your lot and treat a problem. The key is getting to know and understand your skin, so that you are able to identify what needs to be done. Make a habit of checking your skin regularly. If you tend to problem skin, be aware of your diet and lifestyle choices – they may well be the underlying cause. Also realize and accept that your skin is constantly changing and that you may need to adapt your skincare routine accordingly.

Histamines are chemicals in your body's tissues. When released, they cause an allergic reaction, which is your body's way of trying to expel a perceived invader.

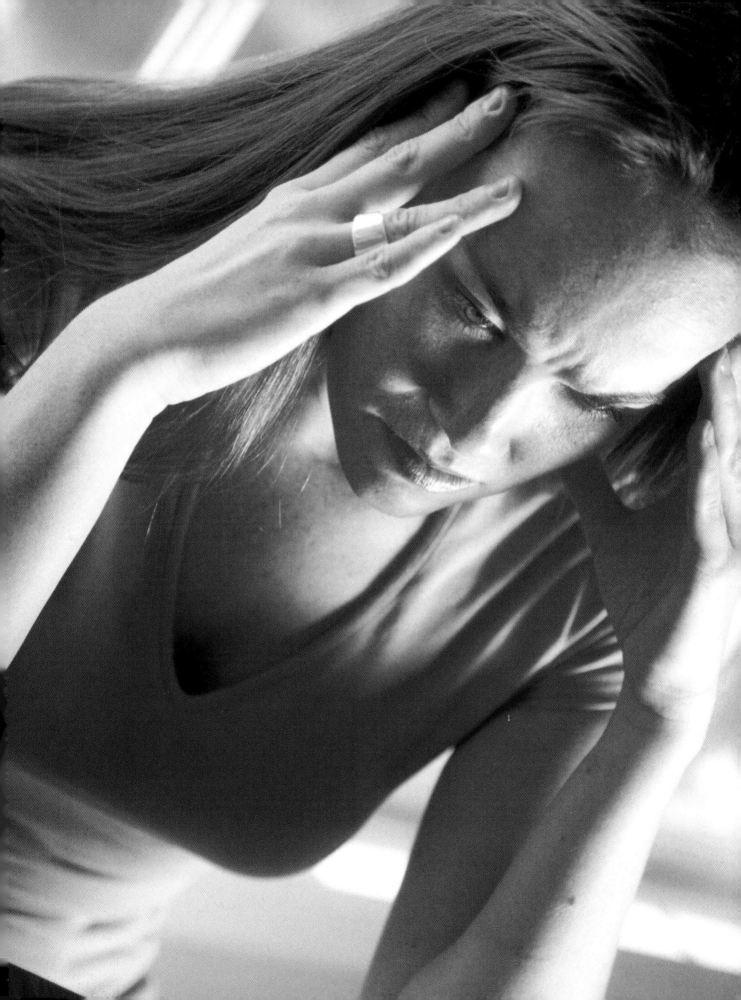

All about acne

Age is not a sure guarantee against pimples or acne. In fact, many people only experience acne for the first time in their adult years; recent studies show that 40–50% of adults between the ages of 20–40 are diagnosed with low-grade persistent acne.

The exact cause of acne cannot be pinpointed. A number of factors seem to have an effect, including genetics, hormones, physiology, stress and the use of certain cosmetics. This type of acne ranges from a few isolated spots to severe breakouts, which can leave unsightly scars. Acne results when the sebaceous (oil) glands secrete too much sebum into the hair follicle, which is lined with dead cells. The combination of excess sebum and dead cells clog up the pores, which are the pipelines for the natural flow of oil to the skin's surface. As a result bacteria build up, the area becomes inflamed, and spots or pimples may appear. Acne most commonly occurs where the sebaceous glands are most active – on the face, neck, chest and back. A variety of blemishes result:

- **Whiteheads** form when oil and dead cells accumulate and block the pores from opening onto the surface of the skin.
- **Blackheads** are similar to whiteheads, except the blocked material protrudes above the skin, dilating the pore. The black colour is due to the oxidization process that occurs within the follicle.

◀

If left alone, blackheads will simply stay in the skin. Remove them by gently steaming the area and then 'easing' the plug out.

CROSS SECTION OF A BLACKHEAD

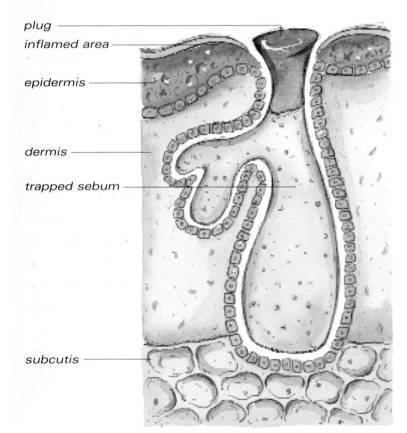

plug

inflamed area

epidermis

dermis

trapped sebum

subcutis

- **Papules** are inflammations under the skin. When the sebum build-up becomes too much, the follicle expands and eventually bursts, releasing the sebum and dead cell build-up onto the surface of the skin. White blood cells then attack this material, forming pus, and a pustule results.
- **Cysts** occur when inflammation spreads deep into the skin. To contain it, the cells automatically form a fibrous capsule around it. Cysts can continue to grow slowly under the skin and usually need to be surgically removed.
- **Scars** result when damaged skin tries to heal itself. Naturally, scars can be severely aggravated by picking or squeezing.

Don't be tempted to remove skin impurities such as blackheads by harsh squeezing or without preparing your skin first.

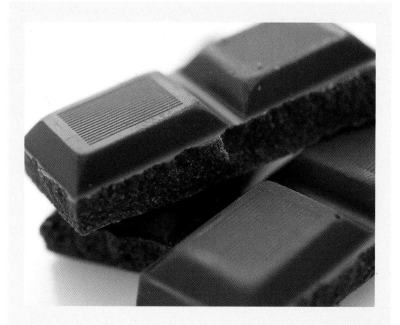

FACT OR FICTION?

Chocolate and fatty foods cause acne. There is no scientific evidence to indicate that diet plays a determining role. The 'westernized' diet is high in preservatives, colourants and processed foods and supports the most acne-prone populations. The Asian and Mediterranean populations, however, generally eat more good fatty acids and far less processed foods. Although acne is less common in these areas, the role of genetic factors is unclear.

Acne is due to poor hygiene. The blackheads we see are a result of an oxidization process that turn the sebum and dead cells black in colour. It is not dirt. In fact, over-cleansing can aggravate acne.

Sunlight improves acne. The sun can seem to improve the complexion, but it also suppresses the immune system. That is why acne often seems to get worse a few weeks after sun exposure. The sun also stimulates sebum secretion. It is more advisable to wear an oil-free sunscreen.

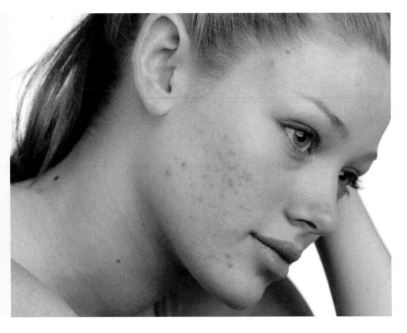

Although more common in teenagers than any other age group, acne can occur at any time in life. The causes are still not completely understood.

◄

Stress inducers include skimping on sleep, skipping meals and ingesting too much caffeine. All these factors trigger the adrenaline in your body to mobilize stored nutrients, which in turn slows down natural exfoliation processes. The remedy? Get enough sleep, follow a balanced diet, drink plenty of water, and cut down on caffeine and high-fat foods. In severe cases or if there is no change, consult a skincare professional.

WHAT CAUSES ACNE?

Hormones

Throughout your life, hormones will play a very important role in determining the ups and downs of your skin. Oestrogen is an important skin regulator, and an excess of male hormones can cause acne. Men and women both produce male hormones (androgen and testosterone) and female hormones (oestrogen and progesterone) – only the ratio of these hormones differ between the sexes. When the levels of androgen increase – during puberty, ovulation, menstruation and childbirth, for example – the skin produces more oil and acne can result.

Diet

There is not enough evidence to suggest that acne and diet are related, but some people find that certain foods make their acne worse. Common culprits include chocolate, caffeine, nuts, high-fat and spicy foods, citrus fruits, refined foods, dairy products, and foods with a high iodide content, such as artichokes, seaweed, spinach and shellfish. Certain medications can also cause a flare-up.

Stress

Stress triggers the adrenal glands to release the hormone cortisol, which increases the secretion of sebum.

Did you know? Skin that is irritated by a cleanser or moisturizer reacts by forming a protective layer by adhering more skin cells onto the surface.

TREATING ACNE–PRONE SKIN

The best way to treat acne is by preventing new spots while treating existing ones. It can often be treated effectively with nonprescription, over-the-counter products.

- A regular purifying and cleansing routine will help remove excess sebum on the skin's surface, a breeding ground for bacteria. Try using a daily gentle antibacterial wash to help cleanse bacteria from the skin, combined with a beta hydroxy acid such as salicylic acid, which stimulates the skin's natural exfoliation process. As dead cells become 'unstuck', there is less chance of clogged pores. Salicylic acid also helps to curb an oily shine.

- Even oily skin needs daily moisture. If your skin is very oily, choose a lightweight lotion to replace moisture without adding oil. Make sure the product you buy is oil-free or noncomedogenic, which means it won't block pores. If you wear make-up, look out for foundations that 'mattify' or control oil, as they will help eliminate shine.

- Remember that fingers dipped into shared products increase the risk of contamination. If possible, opt for products that are specially sealed or have pump dispensers.

- Benzoyl peroxide is a fast-zapping, nonprescription ingredient that is particularly effective at speeding up the drying up and peeling of spots. It is available in varying strengths and should be introduced at low concentrations as it can be very drying and may cause allergies.

- If your acne doesn't respond to nonprescription remedies (give it at least six weeks), it's best to go for a medical diagnosis with a dermatologist who can prescribe a stronger formulation. Antibiotics can be taken orally (erythromycin and tetracycline are commonly used) or applied topically. The two other proven acne treatments are Retin-A and Roaccutane. Retin-A is an imitation of retinoic acid, the naturally occurring form of vitamin A found in the skin. Its main action is keratolytic, which means it acts as a peeling agent that loosens dead surface cells. Retin-A is a very powerful drug that only needs to be applied to the acne areas in very small doses. The problem is that retinoic acid can be irritating and drying, and causes increased sensitivity to the sun and any other products applied to the skin. Retinoid isotretinoin (Roaccutane) is a synthetic version of vitamin A that's taken orally once or twice a day for four months. It's extremely effective, but the side effects include dryness and increased skin sensitivity. Very strict birth control needs to be practiced while taking Roaccutane as it can cause major birth defects.

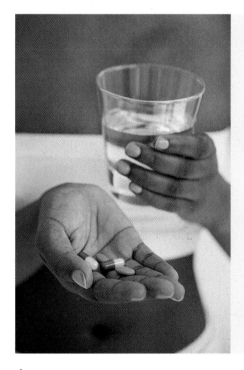

▲

Medication is reserved for more persistant cases of acne and should always be taken under supervision.

Common problems

Eczema generally causes dry and itchy patches of skin.

▼

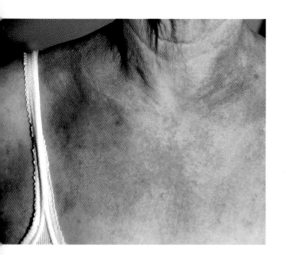

ROSACEA

Rosacea is often referred to as 'acne rosacea' but is not the same as acne. Characterized by red and inflamed skin, particularly on the cheeks, nose, forehead and chin, it may begin as a tendency to blush or flush easily and progresses to persistent redness. Small blood vessels and tiny pimples may also occur. It's most common in women between the ages of 30 and 50 and some cases have been associated with menopause. The exact cause is unknown, although it's believed to be due to a disorder of the blood vessels, which become oversensitive to stimulation. Heat and sunlight may aggravate it as they stimulate the release of chemicals that encourage the blood vessels to enlarge. Rosacea is not caused by excessive alcohol, but can be aggravated by it as alcohol causes the blood vessels to dilate. Severe cases are sometimes accompanied by burning of the eyes. Treatment includes oral and topical antibiotics, good sun protection practices and avoiding extreme temperatures and spicy foods. Cortisone creams may reduce the redness of rosacea, however, they must only be used under the supervision of a dermatologist and for no longer than two weeks at a time as they can thin the skin. Red wine, oranges and caffeine may also aggravate rosacea, as do scrubbing or rubbing the face and irritating facial products. It can become worse without treatment.

ECZEMA

Eczema, also called dermatitis, describes a family of itchy, red skin conditions. Atopic eczema is an illness (usually an allergy) that runs in the family. It is the most common form of eczema and is characterized by chronic dryness, redness, chapping and itching. It usually appears first during childhood and most patients recover before the age of 25, although some live with it their entire lives. It generally runs in families who also suffer from other allergies such as hay fever and asthma. In teens and young adults, the spots usually break out where the elbow bends, on the backs of the knees, ankles, wrists, and on the face, neck and upper chest. It's important not to scratch as this can lead to infection. Atopic eczema can be partly relieved by avoiding irritants like feathers and wool blankets; dogs, birds and cats; harsh detergents; and certain foods such as

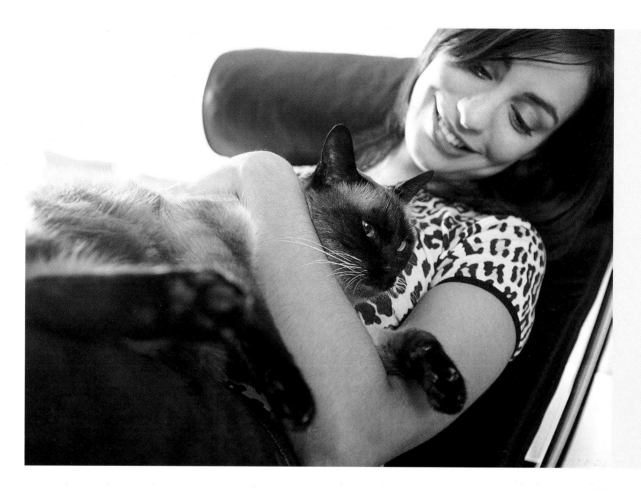

wheat, dairy and chocolate. Stress can also exacerbate the condition. Some over-the-counter products can relieve the itching, while topical steroid creams help soothe and calm the skin. It's best to consult a dermatologist for the correct diagnosis and treatment.

PSORIASIS

This chronic skin disease is caused by an overproduction of cells in the epidermis and ineffective desquamation (shedding of these cells), the combination of which causes cells to accumulate and form red, scaly patches, especially around the elbows, knees, and scalp. Psoriasis tends to run in families and is not contagious. Mild or average cases can be treated with a prescription cream or lotion. If it's severe, your dermatologist may prescribe medication or light therapy. Although psoriasis can be contained, it's unlikely to be permanently cured.

▲

If, unlike this woman, you suffer from atopic dermatitis, you should wash newly bought clothes before wearing them and keep your pets outdoors. Children should avoid fuzzy toys and blankets.

VITILIGO

This skin disease manifests as white patches on the surface of the skin. The patches are due to a loss of pigment, but dermatologists are not entirely sure what causes this.

Vitiligo usually appears on the face, lips, hands, arms, legs and genital areas, but can appear anywhere on the body. The amount of colour a person loses varies: people with a light-coloured skin usually see the difference between patches of vitiligo and tanned skin in summer. For people with darker skin, vitiligo is quite visible all year round.

The most common way to treat it is with light therapy and medicine. It is also possible to hide the marks by using special cosmetic camouflage products. Very often, such products are also water-resistant.

PIGMENTATION

Unbalanced pigmentation is very common and may be a result of years of sun-worshipping or skin trauma.

As discussed previously, the skin has pigment-producing cells called melanocytes that determine skin tone. Dark skins have larger melanin granules, which means more in-built protection, and so are more resistant to sun damage. Fairer skins have less melanin and thus are more likely to develop brown patches from sun exposure. However, skin with more melanin tends to have more hyperpigmentation related to scarring.

While pigmentation can largely be avoided by staying out of the sun, many women experience hyperpigmentation during pregnancy due to hormone activity, even if they avoid the sun. Chloasma or the 'mask of pregnancy' consists of brown patches that appear on the forehead, cheeks and above the lip.

A variety of topical treatments is available that can lighten blemishes, and chemical skin peels, microdermabrasion and laser resurfacing will brighten the skin.

HORMONES AND SKIN

When a woman is pregnant, the additional hormones can cause many changes in the skin. While a beautiful rosy glow is associated with the first trimester and is a result of an abundant supply of oxygen, various sensitivities are likely to appear due to increased hormone activity. Conditions such as rashes, dryness, acne and allergies to your normal skincare products are common.

Did you know? Viruses that sit on the skin's surface and penetrate the stratum corneum when it's damaged cause warts. They can be passed from person to person and are most common on the fingers and feet.

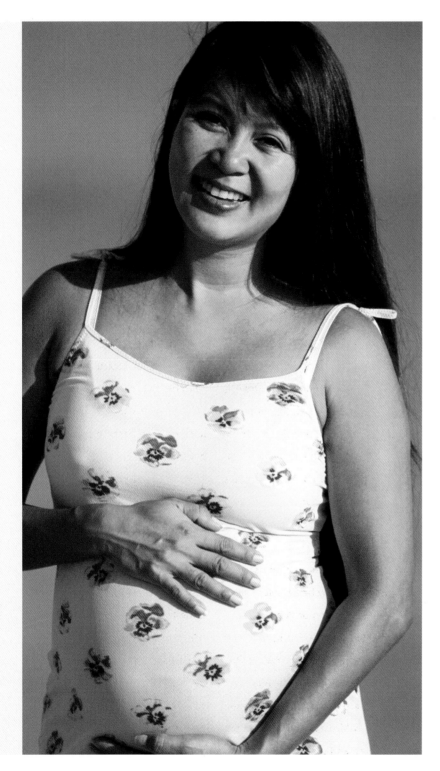

It's important to be extra conscientious with sun protection during pregnancy, as hormonal changes make the skin more susceptible to pigmentation damage. Vitamin supplements are also very important for the maintenance of your skin during this time: vitamin E and zinc have been shown to help reduce stretch marks, and vitamin C aids in collagen production. Always consult your doctor before taking any tablets during pregnancy and while breastfeeding.

Oral contraceptives have similar effects, leading to many of the same skin problems. Although different from person to person, many women on oral contraceptives are more sensitive to sunlight and can develop uneven skin tone and hyperpigmentation if they don't protect themselves adequately. Oral contraceptives can also lead to increased oil production or dehydration.

◀

Pregnancy causes severe hormonal changes in a woman's body that may also affect her skin.

Smoothing the surface

As we age, our faces begin to show the effects of gravity, sun exposure and years of facial muscle movement. Despite the slew of products and advanced technology available today, there is only so much we can do to curb this. Dramatic results can be achieved with face-lifts and reshaping, but there are less-invasive rejuvenating techniques like freezing, filling and polishing. While one needs to accept the inevitable changes that come with age, there is no reason why one should not make use of the sophisticated cosmetic procedures and techniques available. There are so many options, however, that you will need to do some homework. All surgery carries some risk and even less-invasive techniques can have side-effects. Use reputable, certified professionals. Get recommendations or contact the dermatological or plastic surgeons association in your country. Know what can and can't be improved and allow for recovery time. There are quick procedures such as 'lunch-time peels', while other treatments leave your skin red and inflamed for a few days and will require some time off.

Though surgery can have dramatic results, remember that beauty really does start within. Look after what you have and celebrate your uniqueness.

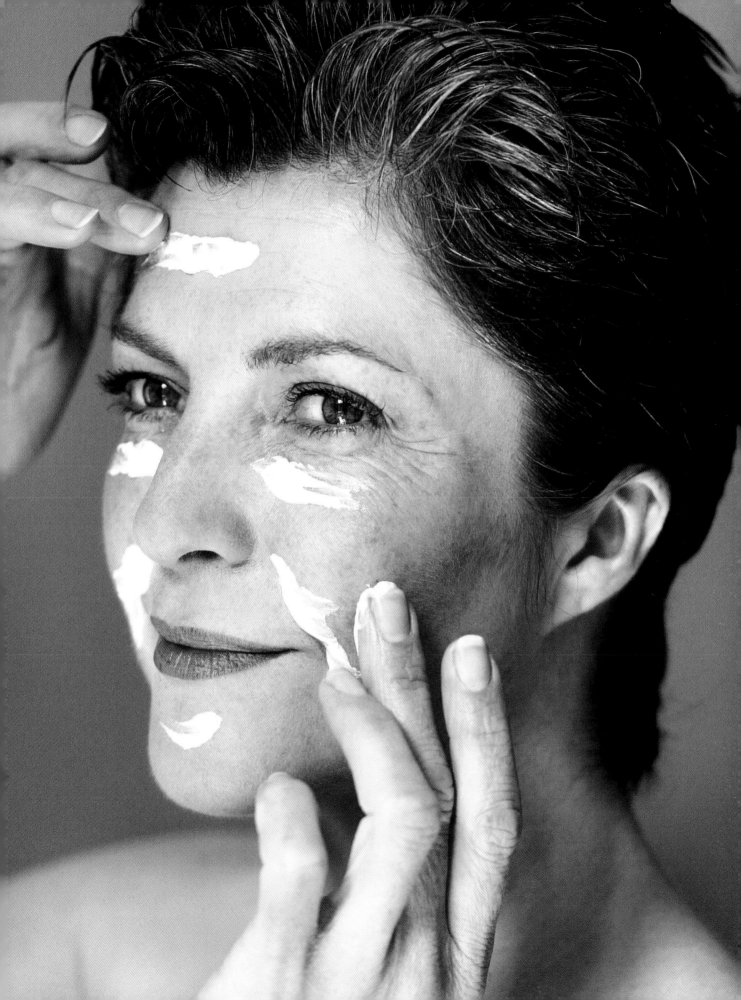

Botox injections have become a popular lunch-time fix; other than the possibility of some redness and very slight swelling at the site, patients can immediately resume their activities.

Whatever method you choose to rejuvenate your face, you should aim to create natural-looking results. Always consult a registered dermatologist or plastic surgeon, and be realistic about what the procedures can and cannot achieve.

There are three types of wrinkles. Static wrinkles are with you all the time, even when your face is at rest. Dynamic wrinkles are created by your facial expressions, and folds are lines that develop when the skin loses its youthful elasticity and begins to sag. Examples of the latter include droopy eyebrows, bags below the eyes, jowls and nasolabial folds (between the corners of your mouth and the sides of the nose). Various non-invasive techniques can help to improve these and they can be used in conjunction with surgery.

FREEZERS

Botox has become the treatment of choice to get rid of expression lines – those that form when your frown, smile or laugh. Botox is a neurotoxin produced from the botulinum bacteria. When injected into a muscle, it acts as a nerve impulse blocker, temporarily paralyzing the muscles and so keeping them from contracting.

Because it 'freezes' the expression muscles, your ability to move the muscle temporarily disappears along with the wrinkles. Botox is most effective on frown lines, forehead lines and crow's feet (on the outer corners of the eyes). The procedure is painless – just a needle prick, but a topical anaesthetic cream can be used if the client prefers or if multiple sites are planned. The procedure takes about 10 minutes and the effect takes four days to a week to kick in. It lasts from three to six months and must be repeated to maintain results. Injections can cause redness and swelling at the injection site and it's advisable not to do anything too strenuous on the day of treatment; nonetheless you can go about your business almost immediately. In rare cases, Botox injections too close to the eyelid muscles can cause the eye area to droop temporarily.

FILLERS

Soft-fillers are injected into the skin to fill lines and wrinkles and build or plump up areas like the lips and cheeks. There are temporary and permanent fillers, as well as exogenous (foreign substances such as collagen) and autologous (one's own tissue or fat) implants. The fat-injection procedure involves extracting fat cells from the patient's abdomen, thighs, buttocks or elsewhere, and re-injecting them beneath the facial skin. This method is usually used to fill in cheeks and lips or to fill laugh lines between the nose and mouth or on the forehead. As the fat is taken from the person's own body, there is no reaction because the immune system immediately recognizes the tissue.

The disadvantages of foreign collagen implants (extracted from cow skin or a human cadaver) are that they only last for two to six months, and that skin testing is required in order to avoid possible allergic reactions.

The more popular temporary filling method is with hyaluronic acid (such as Restylane, Hylaform, Perlane). Hyaluronic acid is a substance that occurs naturally in the skin, so allergic reactions are rare. Injected into the skin in tiny amounts with a very thin needle, the gel adds natural volume under the wrinkle. The product is biodegradable and so will gradually be absorbed. As the gel breaks down, water takes its place and when it is totally absorbed, the gel disappears unnoticed from the body. The procedure takes up to half an hour.

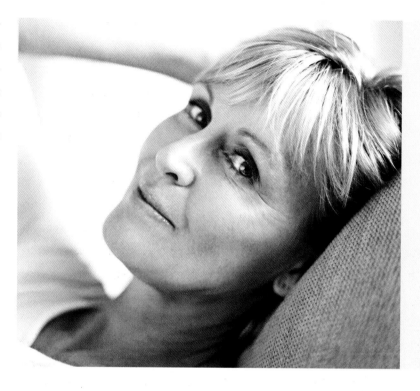

After the treatment you could experience some swelling, tenderness and redness, but these symptoms will disappear in two to four days. How long the effect lasts depends on the individual, but it is generally effective for up to six months after lip augmentation, and up to 12 months after facial contouring.

Other filler materials being used include Fibril, a gelatin powder compound that's mixed with the patient's own blood and is injected to plump up the skin; GORE-TEX®, a thread-like material that is implanted beneath the skin to add soft-tissue

▲

Invasive rejuvenation treatments can tax the body. Regard them as you would minor surgery and allow your system enough time to recuperate.

support; and Zyderm (a bovine collagen) and Zyplast (a cross-linked form of collagen), which are used to improve the appearance of wrinkles, scars and to add volume to the lips. Injectable fillers are not permanent and the body will eventually process the injected material. How long it lasts differs from person to person.

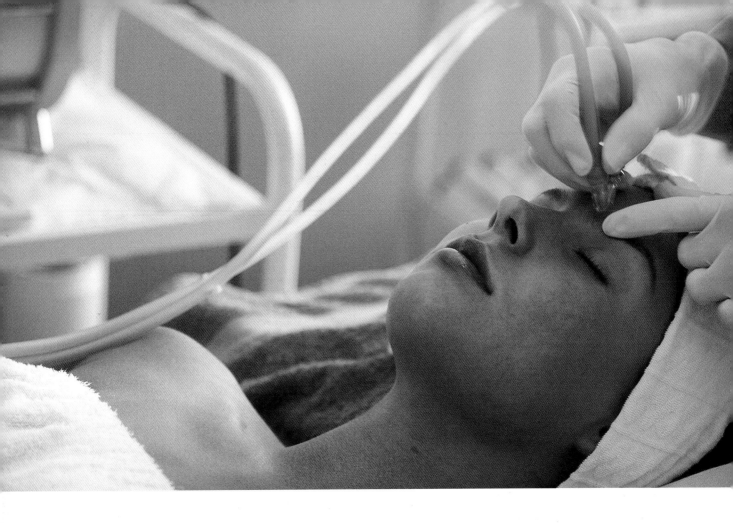

MICRODERMABRASION

Often referred to as the 'lunch-time peel', microdermabrasion is a skin polishing technique that uses microparticles to abrade and rub off the top skin layer, removing the particles of dead skin to give it a smoother appearance. The operator uses a handheld device that blasts fine particles of sand-like crystals (aluminum oxide or table salt) against the skin and vacuums away the used crystals, dirt and dead surface skin. It takes only 20 to 30 minutes for a full-face treatment and can also be used on the neck and chest.

There may be mild redness, which can be covered up with makeup and fades after a couple of hours. This procedure is not painful (there may be a slight tingling) and won't lighten or darken black skin as some strong exfoliating treatments do. It's recommended for smoothing away roughness, fine lines, sun-damaged or pigmented skin, age spots, scarring from acne, accidents or previous surgery, and even precancerous growths. Microdermabrasion exfoliates skin faster and more efficiently than any salon facial and penetrates the skin

All invasive skincare procedures carry some risk. It is vital to consult a registered skincare professional and ensure you are getting the right treatment for your particular concern.

more deeply than a glycolic acid peel. It is not recommended as a treatment for crow's feet because, if used too close to the eyes, the crystals can cause eye irritation and the delicate eyelid skin can be damaged by the machine's suction.

INTENSE PULSED LIGHT THERAPY (IPL)

A fairly new, convenient and thus increasingly popular alternative to laser skin resurfacing and chemical peeling is the use of intense pulsed light. With this type of therapy, an intensive light source is directed towards the surface of the skin. It spreads in all directions and there is no danger of burning or scarring as there is with regular laser.

This therapy is particularly effective for rejuvenating the skin, not just superficially but in the deeper levels, too. The light pulses are adjustable in wavelength and duration so that a variety of tasks can be performed and objectives achieved.

Intense pulsed light therapy helps to improve redness (it's particularly effective in the treatment of rosacea); reduce broken capillaries, brown spots, UV damage, fine wrinkles and large pores. It can even out skin tone and firm the skin. One of its biggest advantages is that there is no down time. Each treatment takes approximately 20 minutes and patients can return to their daily activities immediately afterwards. There is also minimal discomfort – no anaesthesia or topical anaesthetic cream is needed.

This, coupled with an absence of scars and ease of treatment, makes an attractive number of advantages over laser skin resurfacing, chemical peeling, or microdermabrasion. Aftercare is customized to each patient's individual skin sensitivity. This rejuvenation technology is certainly cutting edge and very exciting. As with all of these procedures, it must only be administered by a skilled and qualified professional and a series of treatment is recommended to get the best possible results.

IPL is a fairly recent skin rejuvenation technique that is quick, painless and without any of the nasty side-effects that accompany the other, more invasive procedures.

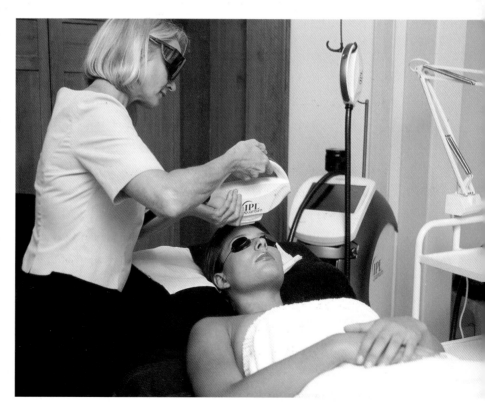

Age, gravity, sun exposure, smoking and stress changes the way a face looks. Creases form and it begins to lose its youthful definition.

▼

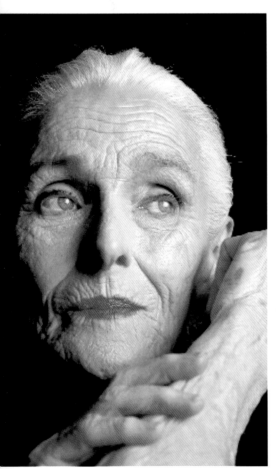

CHEMICAL SKIN PEELS

These peels use a chemical solution to smooth the texture of the skin by removing the damaged outer layers. There are various kinds available. Alpha hydroxy acids such as glycolic, lactic or fruit acids are usually the mildest of the formulas. They can be used to remove the top layer of skin to treat fine lines, even out skin tone and uneven pigmentation and smooth acne scars. They also stimulate cell metabolism, increasing the skin's natural functions. The process takes about 10 minutes. The cons: it can irritate the skin, and you have to undergo a series of treatments to reap the benefits.

Trichloroacetic acid (TCA) is most commonly used for medium-depth peeling to smooth out fine surface wrinkles, blemishes and uneven pigmentation problems. The treatment takes 10 to 15 minutes and can be used on the neck and body. Although healing is quicker than a phenol peel, the results are usually less dramatic and not as long lasting. Repeated treatments may be needed to maintain results.

Phenol is the strongest of the chemical solutions and is used mainly to treat patients with deep wrinkles, sun-damaged skin or precancerous growths on the face. It's more suitable for fair skins as there is a high risk of loss of pigment. A full-face treatment may take an hour or more.

Recovery is slow, complete healing sometimes taking several months. Although the results are dramatic and can last for decades, your skin will never tan again and extreme caution must be taken in the sun.

LASER RESURFACING

Laser facial resurfacing (laser peeling) can be used to smooth skin at almost any age. The top layer of skin is peeled away while the collagen underneath is thickened and re-formed. When your skin heals, it looks brighter and plumper. Laser works well on sun-damaged skin, brown spots, fine lines and veins. It doesn't improve sagging and so is often recommended in conjunction with a face-lift. Laser resurfacing works by directing an intense beam of laser light back and forth over the area being treated. Each pass of the light vaporizes the upper layers of damaged skin and causes the skin to contract. This results in tightening of the collagen and elastic fibres of the dermis, producing a new skin layer that is tighter, firmer and more youthful looking. There are many types of lasers: CO2 and erbium are among the more popular ones. The CO2 is the most aggressive (and effective) treatment for skin that is severely aged or scarred. It is essentially a powerful beam of light that vaporizes the top layers of the skin on contact, prompting it to rebuild itself from the bottom up. It can take from 10 minutes to more than an hour, and must always be performed by a qualified surgeon.

Recovery takes about 10 days, during which time the skin is very swollen, raw and oozing. Crusts form that will eventually fall off. There will be pain, similar to that of severe sunburn, for a few days. Because of the risk of hyperpigmentation, this type of laser treatment is not recommended for darker skin.

The erbium also vaporizes the outer layers of skin, but it resurfaces with less heat, so healing takes place in about a week, with most redness fading within 7–14 days. This type of laser is good for wrinkles, acne scars, sun damage, and irregular pigmentation, but not quite as effective as the CO2. It is, however, much gentler, has fewer side effects, requires a shorter recovery period and can be used on dark skins.

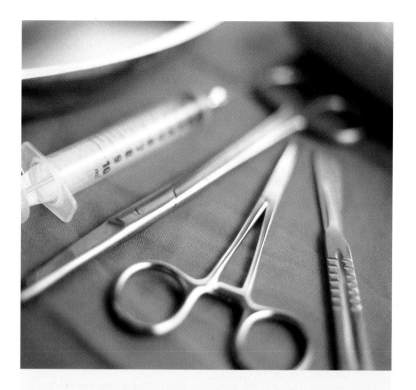

IS SURGERY FOR YOU?

There is no doubt that a face-lift or liposculpture can make an enormous difference not only to a person's face, but also to their self-esteem. If you choose plastic surgery, then follow this advice:

• Be sure of your decision.

• Go to a qualified and reputable surgeon with whom you feel comfortable.

• Be realistic in your expectations. Resurfacing and Botox will improve the overall appearance of your skin's quality; surgery deals with skin quantity and can be used to elevate and reshape sagging contours.

• Get clear answers to all your questions.

• Be aware of the risks associated with surgery.

• Know the full cost and be aware of all the implications before you commit.

• Look after your face and body prior to surgery and follow all post-operative instructions.

Taking care of your body

Your face is exposed and the very first thing people notice, so it generally receives a lot more attention than the rest of your body. And when the focus is shifted to the body, it's usually about losing weight and trying to cover up flaws, rather than celebrating it. But to feel good in your skin, you need to shower as much attention on your body as you do on your face – protecting and caring for the skin, which reacts and changes just as facial skin does. It's also a good idea to listen to your body. Aching muscles, tiredness and stiff joints may be an indication that your body is run down and needs attention. A healthy diet and a fitness regime are essential to keep in shape, but caring for your body is just as much about keeping the skin smooth and glowing with energy. Taking a brisk walk, treating yourself to a long bath or a massage, regular exfoliation, nourishing lotions, keeping an eye on posture, proper breathing and taking time to relax all have a direct impact on your body and its appearance. In this chapter we look at how to keep the body's skin smooth, supple and healthy.

Detoxifying, firming body wraps relieve water retention, making the skin appear smoother. The effect lasts about 8-12 hours.

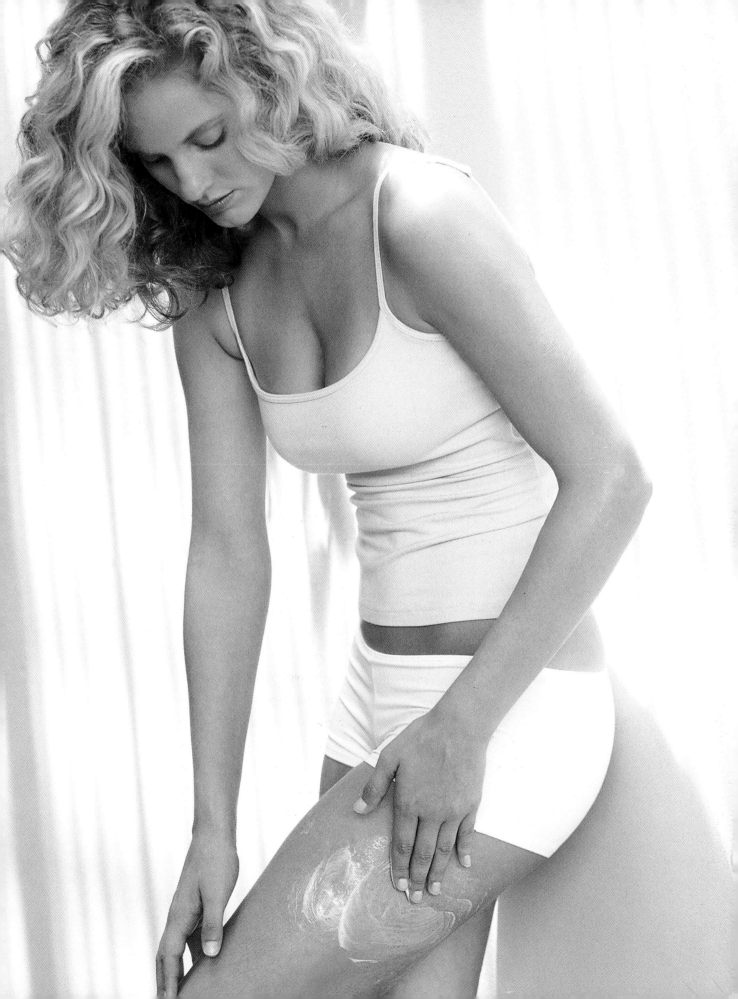

Body basics

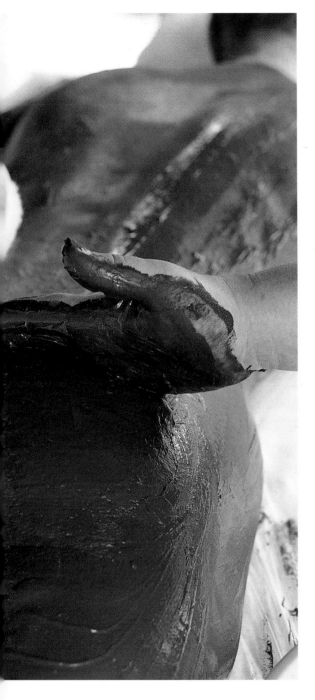

EXFOLIATION

Dry skin is simply the accumulation of dead skin cells. By removing them through exfoliation, skin looks smoother and more youthful; it also helps prevent ingrown hairs. You can either use an exfoliating scrub or a body brush, rubbing gently in a circular motion, towards the heart.

MOISTURIZING

The skin on your body is generally drier than the skin on your face, so daily moisturizing is essential. When choosing a product, remember that the heavier the consistency, the more moisturizing it is. If you suffer from spots on your chest or back, look for a body lotion that contains salicylic acid. Many lotions also contain AHAs, retinol, antioxidants and sunscreens, so you really can give your body the same attention as you do your face. Apply it immediately after bathing to seal in the moisture.

HAIR REMOVAL

Unwanted hair can be removed in a variety of ways depending on your time and pain threshold! And, various lotions can be applied after your method of hair removal to inhibit regrowth.

- **Depilatories** are creams and lotions that contain chemicals to dissolve hair. They can irritate the skin whose outer layer is made of a keratin protein similar to that of hair. They are also very alkaline and so can disturb the skin's natural pH balance. Always

Why do ingrown hairs form?

An ingrown hair is a hair that has grown sideways, forcing the tip of the hair into the follicle wall. It can also occur if the hair is too weak to push through the follicle. Regular exfoliation will help reduce the occurrence, while a cream containing benzoyl peroxide, salicylic or glycolic acid can be dabbed on to clear it up.

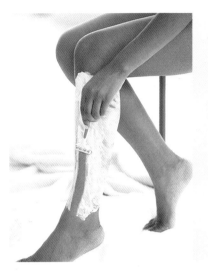 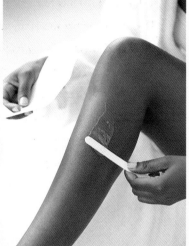 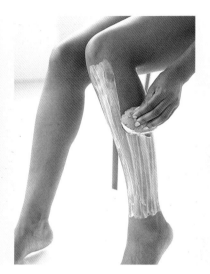

do a patch test first, and never leave on longer than instructed.

• **Shaving** is quick and convenient in the bath or shower. First wash the area with warm water to avoid razor burn and soften the hairs. For minimal irritation, change the blades regularly and use the fewest possible number of strokes. Shaving creams, gels and lotions provide a layer of protection by increasing lubrication so the blade glides smoothly. Most of them also contain soothing and moisturizing ingredients. If you do suffer skin sensitivity, do a patch test before using one of these products. Despite popular belief, shaving does not make the hair grow back thicker – it's merely the blunt edge as

it grows out that makes it appear a little thicker.

• **Waxing** pulls the hair out from the root. Hairs grow back slower than with shaving and become finer with repeated use. For optimal results, hair needs to be quite long and the process can be painful. Like shaving, waxing can cause ingrown hairs, so exfoliate the area well.

• **Electrolysis**, when it is performed properly, can permanently remove unwanted hair. Electrical impulses are directed into hair follicles where they shock the hair's root and inhibit growth. The procedure is time-consuming and expensive because multiple treatments are required. It can also be quite painful, but an anaesthetic cream can be used to

▲

Shaving, waxing or depilatories ... how you remove unwanted hair depends on personal preference – and your pain threshold.

ease any discomfort. It's important to have it done by a professional as it can leave brown marks or scars if done incorrectly.

• **Laser hair removal** temporarily inactivates the hair follicle. Once the follicle is destroyed, it usually stops producing hair. As with electrolysis, more than one treatment is required and it's the most expensive procedure. A session leaves the area free of hair for four to six weeks. Eventually hair becomes finer or disappears altogether.

71

All about cellulite

Cellulite is the dimpling of the fatty tissue under the skin and anyone can have it, no matter how over or under-weight you are. Some experts believe it's a result of genetic, circulatory and metabolic factors, and say there are ways to at least improve its appearance. Others say it's purely an accumulation of fat and no amount of body brushing or expensive potions will disperse it. Another line of thinking is that it's a build-up of fat and toxins like lymphatic fluids, acidic waste and water, due to bad habits such as a sedentary lifestyle, poor diet, alcohol and smoking. This school of thought advocates massage or some other form of stimulation to flush out the nasty stuff.

The most accepted explanation is that cellulite is a woman's condition that's related to oestrogen, the female hormone, which kicks in at puberty and creates curves by enlarging the fat cells, especially on the hips and thighs. The appearance of cellulite is caused by the way a woman's fat cells are packaged underneath the skin: standing chambers of fat separated by fibrous membranes. As we age, the connective tissue between these chambers thickens, causing a mattress-like effect. As the skin thins and fat deposits increase, so the 'mattress' is more exposed. Although it's difficult to get rid of cellulite completely, there are four types of treatments that have shown varying degrees of success.

- **Creams and lotions** are being produced in the thousands, with all sorts of claims to reduce and remove cellulite. The ingredients in these creams, such as caffeine, avocado oil, seaweed and yeast extracts, may work temporarily to some extent, but they would need to be used continually for a permanent effect. A number of women report an improvement in cellulite using over-the-counter creams, but at the same time, many do not. Most of them do help to improve the texture and tone of the surface of the skin.
- **Mechanical massage** like Endermologie, a suction massage treatment, has been shown to minimize cellulite. It works by pulling the skin upwards into a set of rollers under a low-pressure vacuum. This is thought to stretch the vertical connective tissue fibres, resulting in a smoother appearance of the skin.

Medium stiff brushes and loofahs are great exfoliants and are also ideal for improving circulation and drainage. Be gentle and stop using them if your skin is irritated.

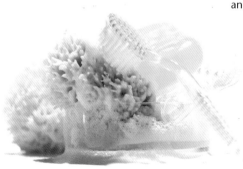

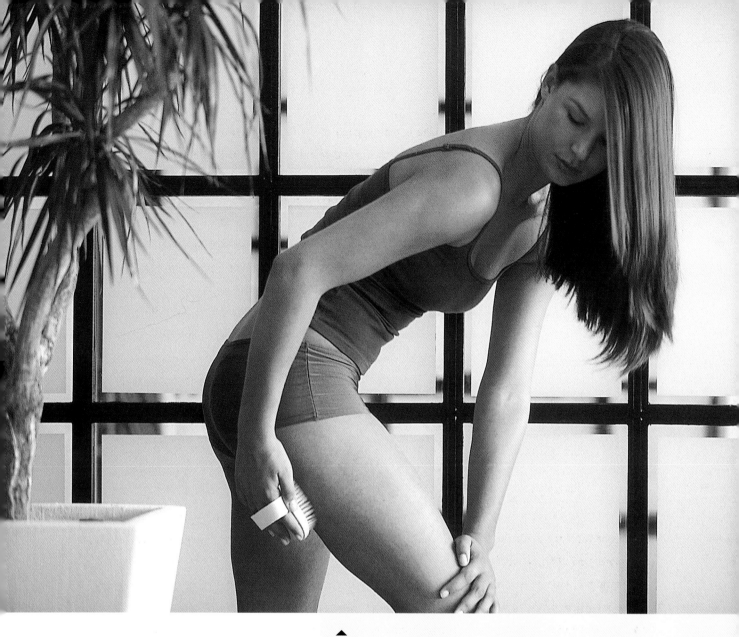

Manual massages such as lymphatic drainage can also help.

- **Diet**, it seems, does not have a direct impact on the formation of cellulite, although crash dieting is a sure way to aggravate cellulite. Every time you restrict calories your body stores fat and reduces muscle and the less muscle you have, the worse your cellulite will be. When you start eating again, it's more likely your body will

Dry body brushing is one of the cheapest and most effective methods of stimulating circulation, which is essential for normal body functioning. If your circulation is impaired, insufficient oxygen and nutrients are delivered to the cells, toxins are not removed efficiently and lymph fluid is not drained correctly.
All this encourages fat and toxin build-up. When body brushing, brush firmly towards the heart, but be careful if you have any problem skin conditions.

73

Why don't men get cellulite?

There are a few reasons why women are the unlucky recipients of the orange peel effect. Firstly, the basis of cellulite is believed to be the female hormone, oestrogen. Secondly, fat is distributed differently in men and women. In women, it's stored mainly in the buttocks and thighs – where cellulite is generally located – and in men in the belly. Thirdly, men and women's fat sacs are packed differently in the skin. A woman's fat cells are standing chambers with the connective 'ropes' pointing up towards the surface, thus creating the dimple-like effect. Men's fat sacs, on the other hand, lie horizontally. The connective tissue is also horizontal and therefore doesn't show on the surface.

gain the weight back as inactive fat, rather than active muscle. A balanced diet and six small meals a day is recommended for general health benefits. Eat the smallest meal in the evening when your metabolism and ability to burn calories is at its lowest. Minimize intake of fatty and refined foods, sugar, dairy, alcohol, caffeine and red meat.

• **Exercise** can also play a role in reducing the appearance of cellulite as it improves your circulation, which in turn burns fat and helps strengthen the connective tissue structure under the skin. The effects of exercise, however, will vary from person to person.

Vein removal

Spider veins are small, dilated blood vessels that appear red or blue under the skin. Until recently, most spider leg veins were treated with sclerotherapy, which involves injecting a solution directly into the vein, causing it to close up and disappear within a few weeks. Though a successful treatment, side effects include skin ulceration, the formation of very fine blood vessels that appear as pink patches, brown staining of the skin, and, rarely, blood clots or allergies to

the solution. Laser technology now allows dermatologists to zap these veins with good results. Several sessions of 10 to 15 minutes each at one to two month intervals are needed in order for the damaged blood vessels to be cleared away by the body's immune system.

Varicose veins are much thicker than spider veins and have a purplish tinge. They usually occur on the legs and are caused by a malfunction of

If you have a tendency to develop leg veins, avoid standing for long periods, wear support hose for varicose veins and exercise regularly. Exercise tones the calf muscles which help propel the blood back to the heart, thus avoiding pooling in the lower legs.

the vein's valves, which can be stretched during pregnancy, or as a result of obesity, blood clots or even a genetic defect. If the valve can't close normally, the blood flows backwards and pools in the vein. There are various ways of treating varicose veins. A saline solution can be injected to restrict expansion of the vein, the vein can be closed at the valve or, in severe cases, the vein can be removed completely. New procedures include a laser fibre that is inserted like a catheter directly into the damaged vein; the laser energy heats and seals the vein from within. Another treatment option uses radiofrequency technology to destroy the vein by heating it from within.

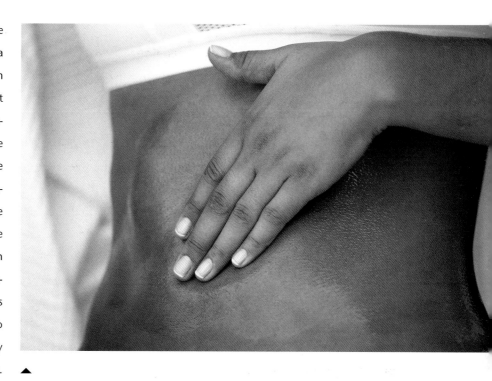

▲

Vitamin E is a perennial skincare favourite and many swear by its healing properties, particularly with regards to preventing and treating stretch marks.

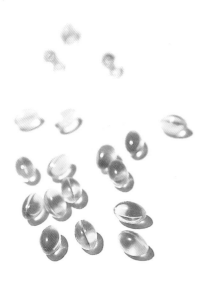

Stretch marks

If skin is seriously overstretched, such as when the body grows faster than the skin can handle (during pregnancy, sudden weight gain, quick muscle-building), collagen fibres in the middle layer can rupture and deep scars can be seen through the epidermis. These are commonly known as stretch marks. While they do fade with time, there is little you can do to get rid of them altogether. Microdermabrasion, laser resurfacing and intense pulsed light treatments may help. Generally, the longer you've had them, the less chance there is of reducing them. Some people swear by vitamin E. It's a good idea to apply vitamin E throughout a pregnancy or if you are trying to lose weight, as it helps keep the skin supple and may therefore help reduce the incidence of stretch marks. Fake tan can help disguise them.

Straighten Up

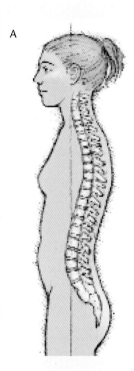

A

No matter what your shape or size, standing up straight will make you look and feel better. In fact, you can look as though you've lost five pounds simply by standing and walking correctly.

Not only does a good posture help to make you look stronger, taller and more graceful, it is also very good for your health as it lessens the chances of back and neck problems, weak stomach muscles, tiredness and poor circulation.

To determine if your posture is good, stand as you usually do, with your heels against a wall. Your calves, buttocks, shoulders and the back of your head should touch the wall and you should just be able to slip your hand between the small of your back and the wall.

If, after doing this little test, you decide that your posture is not what it should be, then here's what you can do to improve it:

• When you're sitting, pull your navel in towards your spine and stretch the torso so it's upright.

• When standing for long periods of time, remember to check that your abdominal muscles are pulled in tight towards your spine, your hips are tilted slightly forward and your knees are relaxed.

• Exercise is a good way to improve your posture. Make sure you are doing exercises correctly, especially if it involves equipment at a gym.

• If you spend a lot of time sitting at a desk, find a chair that supports your lower back and keep your feet flat on the floor.

• To strengthen your back, squeeze your shoulder blades together and hold for 10 seconds. Repeat 10 times. Do this regularly throughout the day.

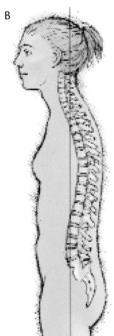

B

▶

Good (A) versus Bad (B).
Not only is a sloppy posture
unattractive, it also restricts your
circulation and limits your breathing.

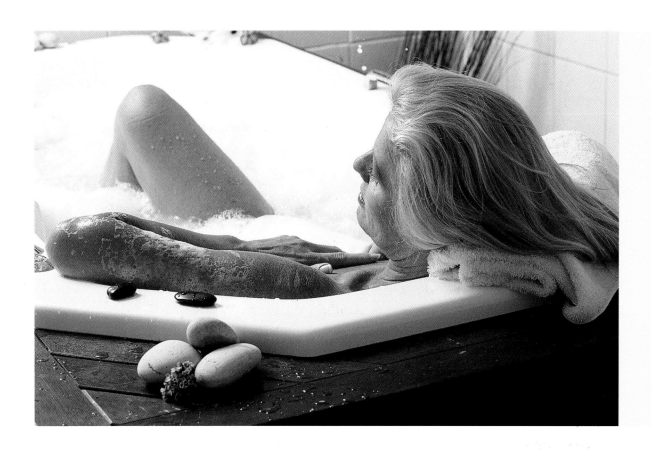

Bath time

A relaxing bath can be a real treat for face and body. To get the most out of it, try these tips:

- The heat of a bath helps to open pores and relieve congestion. If you suffer from spider veins, broken capillaries or flush easily, avoid very hot baths and Jacuzzis.
- Add a few drops of essential oil to the water. You can choose the oil according to the effect you would like to create; relaxing, soothing or invigorating. Focus on the smell of the oil and enjoy it.
- Climb into the bath and take a few moments to unwind. Start by relaxing your neck muscles, then your shoulders, arms, chest, back, tummy, hips, thighs, knees and finally, your feet.
- As you relax, concentrate on your breathing. Inhale deeply through your nose to a count of four, letting the air fill your chest and work its way down into your abdomen. Hold for a count of eight and then exhale slowly through your mouth. Repeat a few times.
- Once you've soaked (keep it to 15 minutes – more than that and your skin will become puffy), wash by rubbing with long, smooth strokes towards the heart.
- When you get out of the water, dry yourself and apply a generous dollop of moisturizing lotion. Alternatively, apply essential oils while the skin is still damp, this will help to seal in moisture.

Feeding your skin

Your skin reflects your state of health. If you follow a healthy, balanced lifestyle, eat sensibly, keep stress in check and allow enough time to pamper yourself and recharge your batteries, you are less likely to suffer the skin diseases and disorders discussed in previous chapters. If, on the other hand, you subject your body to all the things we are told not to do (smoking, poor diet, lack of exercise and overload at work), the chances are you're not going to look as good as you could after a few months. The warnings are unmistakable, but it is important to remain realistic about one's lifestyle: there is only so much each of us can do to try and reduce stress levels; apart from recycling and trying to contribute as little as possible to pollution, there's very little we can do about it, and it is not always easy to give our bodies exactly the fuel that they need. The key is to try to live as vibrantly as possible. Supplement to replace missing nutrients, take time out when you need it and have fun. It's all about making an effort to live well, because that is your insurance for good health and great skin.

Relaxed breathing and elevated concentration levels will help you to lower your heart rate and blood pressure and increase your peace of mind.

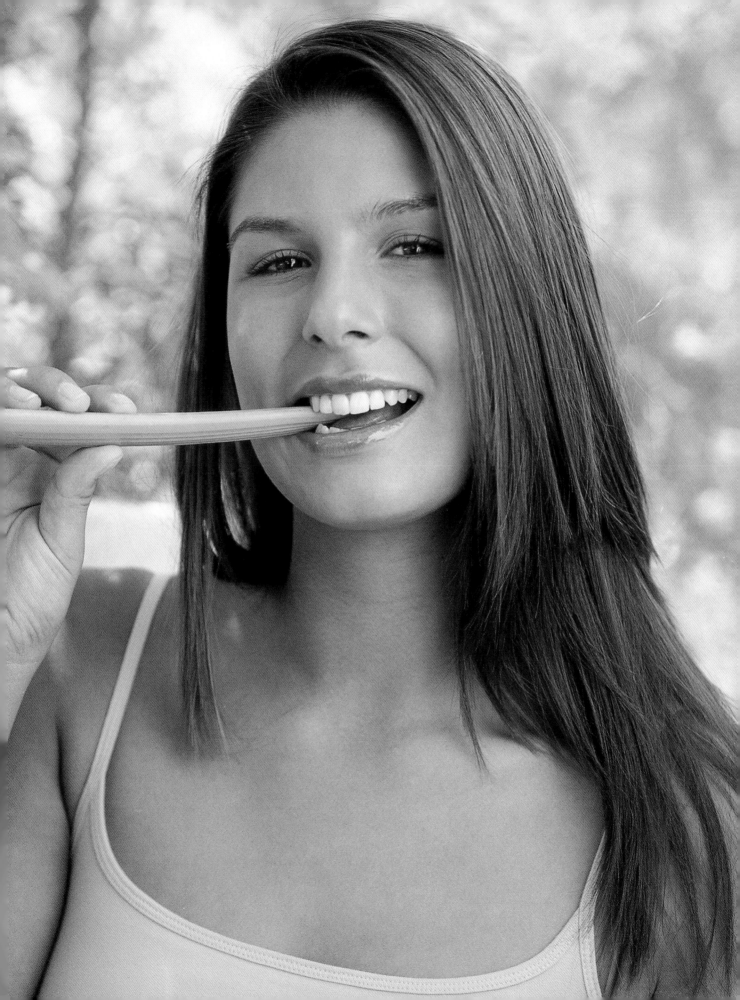

The stress index

In chapter one we mentioned that stress can make skin behave badly. For some people it takes severe and prolonged stress to reach the breaking point, while for others it may only take smaller irritations like traffic jams, having to do a presentation, or lack of sleep to induce a physical or emotional outbreak. Short-term stress is beneficial in that it prepares the body for an emergency. However, in the long-term, your body, skin and health start to suffer. Unlike other hormones, cortisol – the stress hormone – does not decrease with age. In a young, healthy body, cortisol levels increase in the morning and drop at night. If you are under prolonged stress, cortisol is continually secreted into the bloodstream. A younger person is more able to move from a stressed

▶

As little as two cups of coffee a day can dramatically increase levels of cortisol – the stress hormone – in your body.

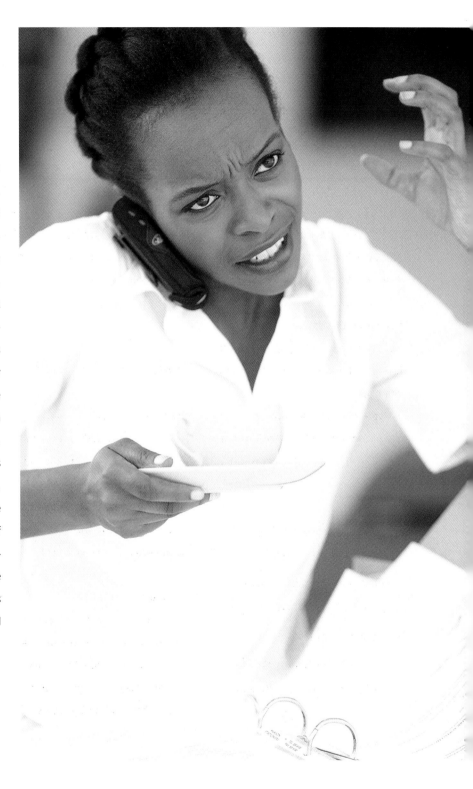

state to a relaxed one, whereas with age, this becomes more difficult. Problems arise when the body makes too much cortisol for too long. Effects include inflammation – a major contributor to skin ageing, weakening of the immune system and increasing blood sugar levels.

Long-term stress also depresses DHEA, an important steroid hormone for the skin. High cortisol and low DHEA levels are associated with rapid skin ageing. In order to protect the body from the effects of stress therefore, you need to keep your cortisol levels in check. Doing the following can help:

• Eat a diet high in raw and fresh fruits and vegetables. Stick to low glycaemic fruits like citrus fruits (oranges, grapefruit, limes, lemons), deciduous fruits (apples, cherries, peaches, apricots, nectarines, plums, pears, strawberries), kiwifruit and grapes. They help to detox the body, balance hormones and increase levels of potassium – which is essential for beautiful skin.

• Get enough exercise.

• Watch your vitamin intake. Pantothenic acid, vitamins B6 and C, zinc and magnesium support adrenal function and you should get enough of all of them.

Eat at least five servings of fruit and vegetables per day. Wash them thoroughly to remove pesticides.

Relaxed breathing and elevated concentration levels will help you to lower your heart rate and blood pressure and increase your peace of mind.

THE EFFECTS OF STRESS ON THE SKIN

Sallow complexion

Stress sends the body into survival mode by directing most of the blood to the vital organs such as the heart, lungs and brain. This means less blood goes to the skin, which leaves you looking washed out.

Pimples

Cortisol causes the secretion of androgen, a sex hormone that increases oil production. Excess sebum means clogged pores, which then leads to breakouts.

Rough, dry skin

A restricted blood supply to the skin means the cells renew themselves less quickly, leading to dry, flaky skin.

Inflammation

When your body is stressed it often releases histamines, which can cause irritation like itchiness, bumps, rashes and hives. A routine relaxation or meditation session can help reduce these hypersensitive reactions.

Nourishing from the inside out

Good fats

Although low-fat diets generally lead to better health, our skin actually does need some fat. Eating fat is like 'oiling' your body: the right balance of fats will help maintain the skin's surface barrier and protect against loss of moisture, keeping skin smooth, soft and supple. Fats also transport the fat-soluble vitamins A, D, E and K around the body. But in order to achieve these functions, it's important to eat the right fats. 'Bad' fats are the trans fatty acids found in convenience foods such as highly processed polyunsaturated corn, safflower and sunflower oils, and margarine. They promote heart disease, disrupt the hormonal balance and cause the cell walls to lose their capacity to maintain the moisture balance.

The 'good' fats are the essential fatty acids – omega 3, 6 and 9. Omega 3 fats are found in fatty fish (salmon, mackerel, herring, tuna and sardines), walnuts, flax seeds and flaxseed oil. The omega 6 group is found in avocados, nuts and seeds. The omega 3 oils are vitally important to the skin and have great anti-inflammatory properties. (Remember, inflammation is a major cause of skin ageing.) Omega 9 fats are found in extra virgin olive oil. The easiest way

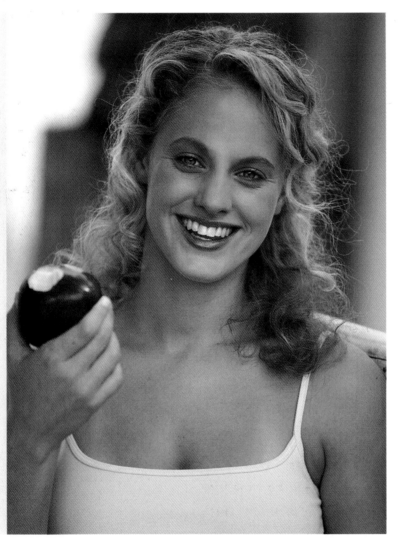

◀

Apples contain minerals such as iron, copper, calcium and magnesium, as well as natural sugars and vitamin C – very good for oily, blemished skin.

to test if you're getting enough EFAs is a simple skin test. Because the skin is the last organ the oil reaches, dry skin tells you that you're not getting enough in. After a hot bath, towel yourself dry and don't apply moisturizer. If your skin feels dry, you need more EFAs. Ideally, you shouldn't need a body lotion because your skin is being lubricated from the inside. EFAs are available in capsule form.

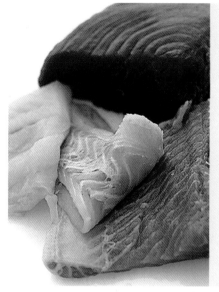

By avoiding junk foods and sticking to a diet that is rich in power foods such as fresh salmon, raw fruit and vegetables, you will soon notice a difference in the appearance and feel of your skin.

The power of protein

Protein is vital for good skin: it contains 25 amino acids – the building blocks of the body – and is essential to build good, strong cell walls. The best proteins come from animal sources – eggs, fish and game meat, and a little from dairy. It is a little more difficult for vegetarians to build beautiful skin, but it is possible. Proteins are also found in dried grains and pulses, like millet, wheat, soy, beans, peas and lentils.

Bright colours

The brighter the colours of your fruits and vegetables, the greater their immune-boosting and antioxidant content. Phytochemicals – natural antioxidants that protect the body against degeneration – are found in bright fruits and vegetables. They support immunity, stabilize vitamins in skin tissues, protect from illness and premature ageing, act as free radical scavengers and help to smooth and firm the skin. The wider the variety of fresh phytonutrient plants you eat, the better.

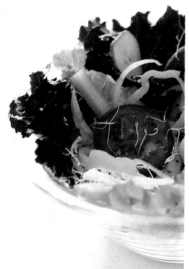

Low sugar

Eating high GI food like bananas, bread, sugar, crisps and cereal, on a regular basis can lead to skin degeneration. You'll see it as loss of radiance, sagging, wrinkles, blotchiness, spots and thin skin. Lower GI foods will help protect your body from blood sugar disorders and insulin resistance syndrome.

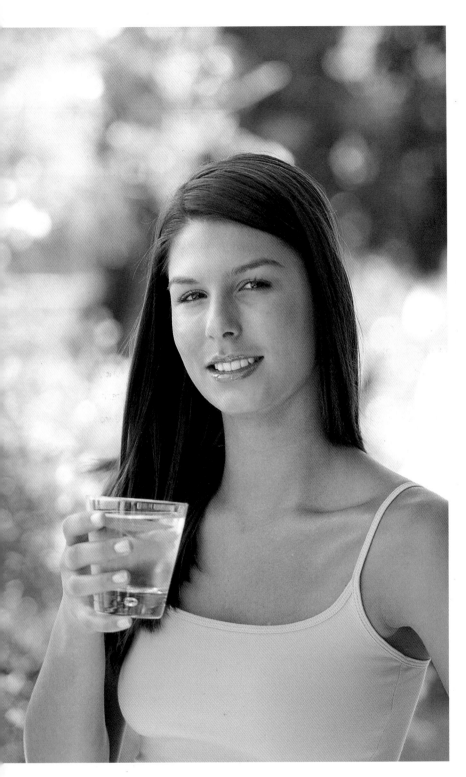

Raw foods

Many nutrients, vitamins and amino acids are destroyed when vegetables are cooked and, in some, the biochemical structure of the nutrients can be altered by heat. The water content is also decreased through cooking. The water found in raw foods is of the highest quality and contains important trace elements, so it's advisable to eat as many vegetables raw as possible.

Water

Water plays a crucial role in digesting your food and absorbing nutrients. If you don't drink enough water, your skin will start to look dry and papery and feel tight. Each time you exhale, you are releasing metabolic waste – about two large glasses a day. Your kidneys and intestines eliminate another six or so glasses every 24 hours and about another two glasses are released through the pores in your skin. On a hot day, this can triple. You need three to four litres of water a day for optimal health. Don't wait until you're thirsty to drink: thirst is a sign that you're already dehydrated.

◀

Your skin is 70% water. If you don't get in your eight glasses a day, your skin can become dry and flaky.

84

CAUSES OF PREMATURE AGEING

Free radicals

Get in enough antioxidants, don't smoke and avoid other forms of pollution as far as possible.

Unstable blood sugar levels

Reduce the amount of carbohydrates in your diet and get enough protein and good fats. Maintain a healthy weight and stop eating when you are 80% full. Eat small, regular meals.

Poor detoxification; sluggish circulation: symptoms include a hung-over feeling (even without the alcohol), chronic fatigue, bad breath, migraines, itching skin, skin allergies, premature photo ageing and pigmentation, joint pains and stiffness, irritable bowel syndrome and chemical sensitivity. Find time to detox, and generally include more healthy food and water in your diet. It's a good idea to visit a health spa to kickstart your detox under supervision.

Chronic inflammation

This is caused by deficiencies of vitamins B6, B12 and folate; a diet high in animal fats; deficiencies of bioflavonoids and antioxidants; food additives, as well as MSG and aspartamine. Increase or reduce these elements as appropriate for your diet.

Impaired immune system function: symptoms include frequent colds, sinusitis, thrush, slow wound healing, recurring bacterial or viral infections. Correct nutrition is essential. Antioxidants, garlic and zinc can help strengthen the immune system.

Prolonged and severe stress

This results in excessive cortisol production, which depresses the immune system and can thus negatively affect other hormones. Find activities that relax your mind and body, and engage in these regularly.

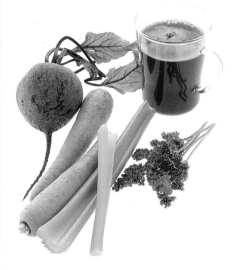

Eat your way to great skin

If you want to look and feel good, supply your body with a few fresh energy foods and it will reward you with glowing good skin:

- freshly squeezed vegetable juice, especially celery, carrot, beetroot and wheat grass
- sprouts and seeds
- red grapes
- yoghurt, fermented foods
- tomatoes, cruciferous vegetables
- garlic, turmeric and ginger
- sardines, salmon and fatty fish
- soy products, tofu
- kelp and seaweed
- olive oil
- blueberries, cherries
- barley grass

Supplements for a healthy skin

- Vitamins A, C and E, selenium and co-enzyme Q10
- The B group of vitamins
- Omega 3 essential fatty acids
- Sulphur (MSM/ methyl sulfonyl methane), a component of cystine that aids in healing and tissue repair. It's necessary to produce collagen and keratin and is useful in treating acne, eczema and psoriasis. It's found in fish, eggs, meat and some fruits and vegetables
- Alpha lipoic acid is a potent antioxidant found in small amounts in animal livers and kidneys, red meat, spinach and potatoes

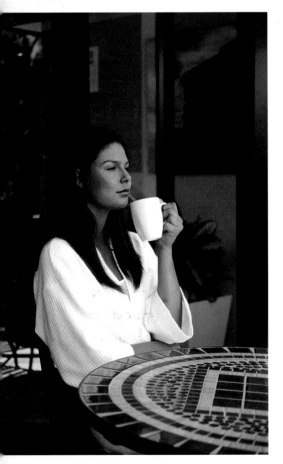

Allow yourself regular 'me' time to relax and reflect.

Relaxation

Taking time to relax is one of the most important things you can do for your health. Less stress not only means fewer frown lines, but deeper health benefits as well, such as improved breathing and circulation and reduced muscle stress.

Meditation

If you battle to switch off and relax, you may want to try meditation. Research shows that regular meditation can help with complaints like headaches, asthma, PMS and hypertension. The idea behind meditation is to empty the mind of all thoughts by focusing on one particular thought. It may be difficult initially, but with practice, you'll find that it becomes easier to slip into a state of calm. Start with five to 10 minutes and increase the time as you feel fit.

- Choose a quiet spot where you won't be interrupted.
- Avoid meditating just before or immediately after a meal. A full or growling stomach is a sure form of distraction.
- Sit comfortably with your hands resting in your lap or lie down. Close your eyes.
- Focus on relaxing one part of your body at a time, starting with your scalp and moving slowly all the way down to your toes. Feel the tension

dissolve from each muscle and each limb, including your face, stomach and back.

- To prevent thoughts of your 'To Do' list or what happened that day at work, focus on one neutral or calming thought. It could be a scene (i.e. the sky), a colour (i.e. blue) or a phrase (i.e. 'I am calm.').

- Let your breathing fall into a natural rhythm. Allow the air to fill your lungs and breathe from the abdomen, not the chest. Inhale through your nose and exhale through your mouth.

- When you are finished, slowly open your eyes and stay quiet for a few more minutes.

If a distracting thought enters your mind while you are trying to meditate, acknowledge it and let it go. Think of it as a balloon floating away into the distance.

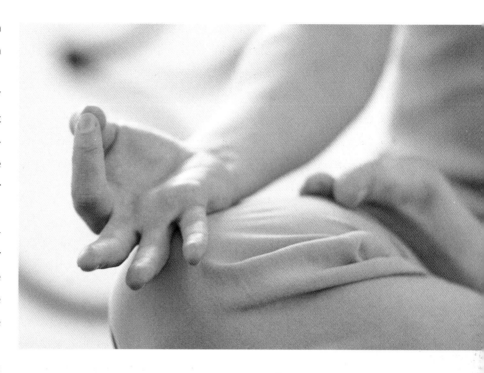

The benefits of meditation

- Cultivates a state of serenity
- Regulates blood pressure
- Activates parasympathetic nervous system, allows muscles to relax and helps regulate breathing
- An effective tool for coping with stress and pressure
- Improves concentration

Breathing

Breathing is linked to our emotions. When we're tense, our breathing is shallow and hurried; when upset, it's irregular; when we're bored, it's long and drawn out. By consciously bringing our breathing under control, we

▲

For total relaxation avoid all other mental stimuli. Within even a couple of minutes you will feel much more clear-headed and rested.

can reduce the effects of emotional turbulence. By refocusing your attention on your breathing, you're effectively pushing the worries out of your mind, and controlled, deep breathing has been shown to aid digestion, oxygenate the brain, alleviate asthma and bronchitis, improve blood circulation and improve the functioning of the immune system.

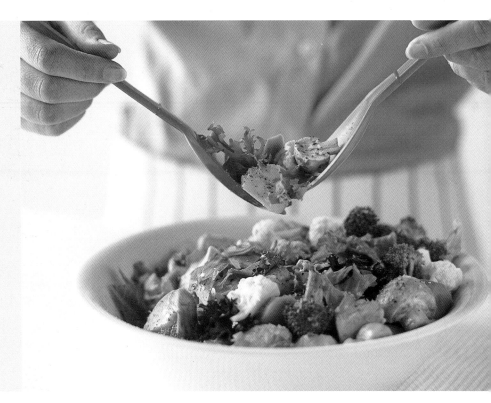

Your body needs to be treated to a regular detox, but there's no need to starve yourself. Brightly coloured fruits and vegetables can be tossed into a salad for a tasty, but healthy lunch.

Weekend detox

We live in a world invaded by toxins, so it's no wonder that our minds and bodies are on toxic overload. One way to combat the negative effects this has on our skin and bodies is to allow for a regular and gentle two-day detox. This gives the body a chance to rest and recharge. After a couple of days of cleansing, you'll feel and look better and can expect a clearer skin, better digestion, heightened senses and possibly even an improvement in illnesses and stiff joints. Always consult your doctor first if you are pregnant, diabetic, on prescription drugs or suffering from illness.

Aim to eat fresh fruits and vegetables and loads of water, avoiding alcohol and caffeine.

- Eat as many fresh and washed fruits for breakfast as you like. Go for low GI, brightly coloured fruits like kiwis, grapes, mango, papaya, peaches, berries, strawberries, pears, apples and nectarines.
- Have a mid-morning snack of a handful of nuts and green tea, herbal tea or plain water.
- For lunch, prepare a power salad containing dark-leaved lettuce, rocket, tomato, cucumber, cauliflower or broccoli, peppers, grated carrot, avocado, wild herbs, onion, radishes and sprouts. Mix a dressing of extra virgin olive oil, chopped herbs, crushed garlic, lemon juice and balsamic vinegar.

- For an afternoon snack, nibble on a handful of sunflower and pumpkin seeds or eat a small carton of plain yoghurt. Sip on a cup of herbal or green tea.
- Dinner can consist of a freshly steamed portion of bright vegetables such as succulent broccoli or cauliflower, leeks, aubergines, onion, marrow, peppers (capsicum), red cabbage, butternut or squash. Flavour with herbs.

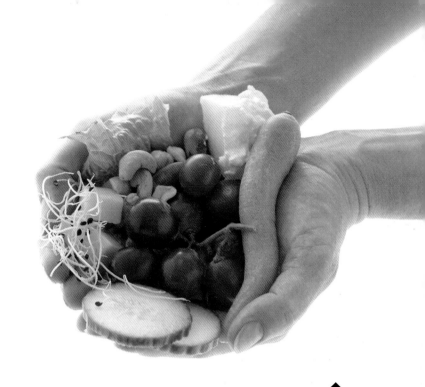

▲

Fresh fruit and vegetables are an instant source of vitamins, fibre, enzymes and antioxidants.

Daily detox

Cleansing from the inside is a very important component if you wish to stay healthy. To help eliminate toxin and fluid build-up, try working the following into your daily routine:

- Drink at least eight glasses of filtered or bottled mineral water a day. If you think it's boring, add a squirt of lemon or lime – they both aid in detoxification.
- Swap your morning cup of coffee for green tea. It's packed with antioxidants and is detoxifying.
- Avoid alcohol. It contains acetaldehyde, which causes the skin to age faster and is also high in empty calories. Hard liquors like whisky, vodka and gin raise insulin levels. However, dry white and red wine do have some antioxidant qualities and may have a beneficial effect; but limit your intake to one or two glasses a day.
- Increase your fruit and vegetable intake. Loaded with fibre and water, they will help to keep your bowels healthy.
- Papaya and pineapple are high in anti-inflammatories and enzymes and aid digestion.

To improve your health, eat fresh vegetables and fruits, as well as enough protein and carbohydrates. A vitamin supplement, at least eight glasses of water a day and regular exercise will keep skin glowing.

89

Home spa

A spa session can be very soothing and revitalizing for the skin as well as for the mind and body. While not everyone can afford the time or money for regular professional pampering, it is fortunately very easy to do a little DIY beauty at home. Try to set aside an afternoon when you're unlikely to be disturbed and give yourself three hours of 'me' time. Spend the time treating your face to a thorough cleanse and gentle exfoliation, nourishing mask and stimulating massage with your fingertips. Give your body the same attention with an invigorating exfoliating scrub followed by a lathering of rich body lotion. As hands and feet are so often neglected, it's also a good time to give yourself a mini manicure and pedicure.

Facial tips:

- To create your own 'steamer', fill a large bowl with very hot water. Hold your head about 15 inches above the water and create a tent by draping a towel over your head and shoulders and the bowl. Stay like this for five to 10 minutes.

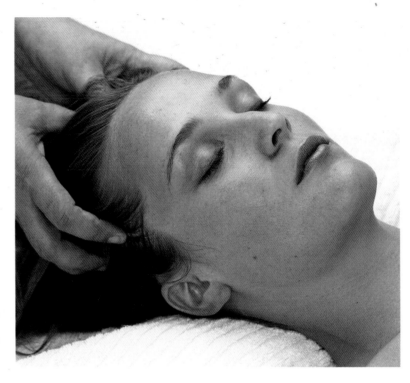

Steaming liquifies the impurities trapped in your pores and helps get rid of blackheads. Avoid this if you're prone to redness or suffer from broken capillaries.

- Choose a mask according to your skin type. If your skin is dry, go for a rich, hydrating product. If it's oily, a clay-based deep-cleansing mask will do the trick.
- You should aim for a salon facial every six weeks or a home regime of gentle exfoliation and a nourishing mask once a week.
- Always make sure your therapist knows your skin's history. If it's

▲

A massage is therapeutic and very relaxing. There are various methods that greatly benefit mind and body.

your first time at a salon, you should be required to fill out a detailed client card.

- The massage action stimulates and oxygenates the skin; the reason skin glows after a facial.
- A facial is also great for reducing stress levels. It forces you to take some time out and relax.

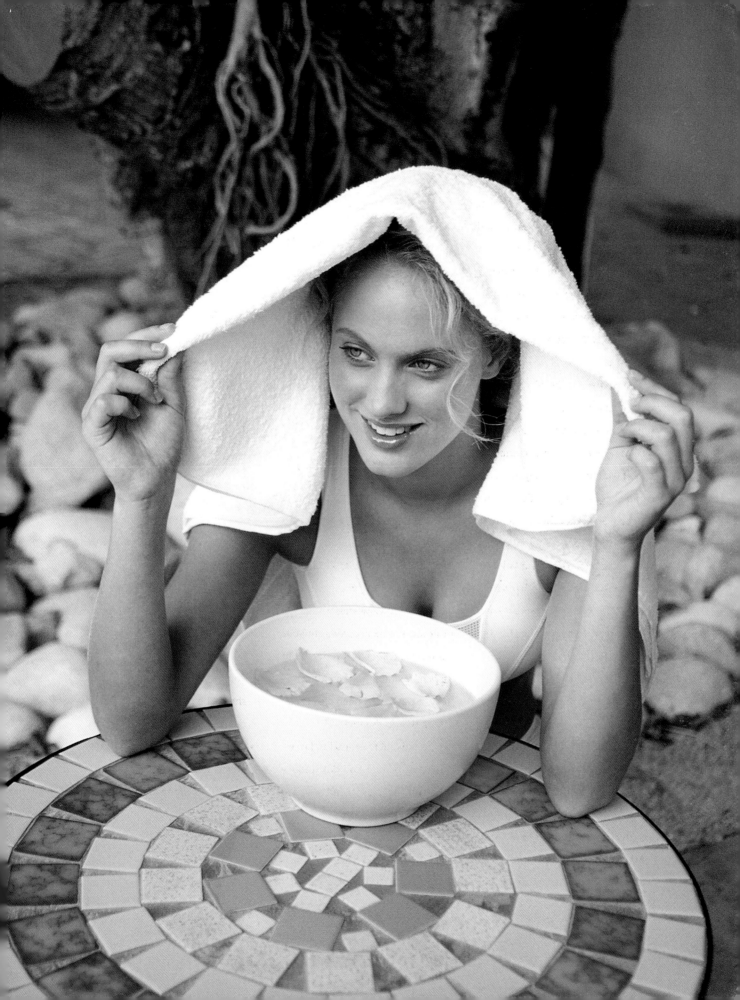

Glossary

ACID MANTLE – protective barrier formed by the stratum corneum and lubricated by the skin's natural oils. Sebum is slightly acidic, hence the name 'acid' mantle.

ACNE – inflammation of the sebaceous glands.

ALPHA HYDROXY ACIDS – also known as fruit acids, this group of natural chemicals is derived from natural ingredients like fruit, olives and milk. They help speed up the exfoliation process by dissolving the glue that bonds the cells.

ALPHA LIPOIC ACID – potent antioxidant found in small amounts in liver, kidneys, as well as red meat, spinach and potatoes.

ANTIOXIDANTS – derived from vitamins A, C and E; part of the body's natural defence system.

ATOPIC ECZEMA – *see* Eczema

BETA HYDROXY ACIDS – natural acids that work in much the same way as AHAs, speeding up cell turnover. The most well known one is salicylic acid.

BLACKHEAD – blockage of sebum and dead skin cells which protrudes above the skin.

BOTOX – neurotoxin which, when injected into a muscle, acts as a nerve impulse blocker, temporarily paralyzing the muscles.

CELLULITE – dimpling of fatty tissue under the skin.

CHEMICAL PEEL – chemical solution to smooth skin texture by removing damaged outer layers.

CHEMICAL SUNSCREENS – cream or lotion that contains synthetic chemical substances which absorb UV radiation.

CO2 – aggressive laser treatment for severely aged or scarred skin.

CO-ENZYME Q10 – occurs naturally in every skin cell and helps convert food into energy.

COLD SORES – *see* Fever blisters

COLLAGEN – protein responsible for the structural support of the skin.

CORTISOL – stress hormone. Prolonged stress causes cortisol to be continually secreted into the bloodstream and can lead to imbalances in the body.

CYSTS – formed when inflammation from a pimple spreads deep into the skin; cysts often need to be surgically removed.

DEPILATORIES – creams and lotions containing certain chemicals that dissolve body hair.

DERMIS – inner layer of skin, beneath epidermis.

DIHYDROXYACETONE (DHA) – colourless sugar in self-tanning lotions that reacts with dead skin cells to create a fake tan.

ECZEMA (also called dermatitis) – skin condition with itchy, red patches. Atopic eczema is the most common type, characterized by chronic dryness, redness, chapping and itching of the skin.

ELASTIN – protein fibres which are responsible for the skin's elasticity.

ELECTROLYSIS – permanent hair removal technique.

ENZYMES – in skincare, botanically derived enzymes that naturally exfoliate the skin.

EPIDERMIS – outer layer of skin.

ERBIUM – laser treatment that vapourizes the outer layers of skin; gentler than the CO2 process.

EXFOLIATION – the process of removing accumulated dead skin cells.

FEVER BLISTERS (also cold sores) – caused by herpes simplex virus.

FIBRIL – gelatin powder compound mixed with the patient's blood and injected to plump up skin.

FILLERS – injected into skin to fill lines and wrinkles and build up areas like lips and cheeks.

FLAVONOIDS – group of organic plant molecules produced by plants to protect themselves.

FREE RADICALS – reactive and unstable molecules, created naturally by the body, which act as scavengers in the skin.

GLYCAEMIC INDEX (GI) – measures amount and rate at which a specific food will raise the blood glucose level.

HISTAMINES – natural chemicals found in the body's tissues. When released, they cause an allergic reaction.

HIVES – localized swellings, usually very itchy, that are caused by the release of histamine.

HUMECTANTS – ingredients that attract moisture from the air to the surface of the skin.

HYALURONIC ACID – natural substance found in the skin, and a popular ingredient in temporary filling methods such as Restylane, Hylaform and Perlane.

LANGERHANS CELLS – found in the epidermis, they protect the body against invaders.

LASER HAIR REMOVAL – temporary inactivation of the hair follicles.

LASER RESURFACING – also known as laser peeling; a method to smooth skin by peeling away the top layer while the collagen underneath is thickened and re-formed.

LIPOSOMES – special microscopic capsules that deliver vitamins directly to the areas needing them most, then release over time for longer-lasting benefits.

MELANOCYTE – melanin producing pigment cell.

MELANOMAS – most widely known and deadliest form of skin cancer.

MINIMAL ERYTHEMA DOSE (MED) – the time it takes for unprotected skin to turn red in the sun.

MICRODERMABRASION – skin polishing technique that uses microparticles to abrade the top layer.

PH – denotes acid balance. Skin is slightly acidic with a pH between 4.5–5.5.

PHYSICAL SUNSCREENS – reflect or block UV rays.

PHYTOCHEMICALS – natural antioxidants that protect the body from degeneration.

PSORIASIS – chronic skin disease caused by the over-production of skin cells in the epidermis, causing red, scaly patches.

RETINOIDS – derivative term for vitamin A.

ROSACEA – condition characterized by red, inflamed skin; may begin as a tendency to blush or flush easily and progress to persistent redness.

SENSITIZED SKIN – skin that has been exposed to an allergen some time in the past and then reacts on each successive exposure to that allergen.

SERUMS – lightweight formulations that have a high concentration of active ingredients and are ideal in caring for temporary skin conditions.

SHINGLES – common skin ailment caused by chicken pox virus.

SPF – Sun Protection Factor, a measure of how much time you can spend in the sun above your MED time.

SPIDER VEINS – small, dilated blood vessels that appear red or blue under the skin.

STRATUM CORNEUM – top layer of the epidermis, also known as the horny layer.

STRETCH MARKS – appear when skin is overstretched, causing collagen fibers in the middle layer to rupture, and forming deep scars under the epidermis.

ULTRAVIOLET RADIATION – a form of sunlight that damages the skin.

VARICOSE VEINS – thicker than spider veins, they have a purplish tinge and are caused by a malfunction of the vein's valves.

VITILIGO – skin disease caused by a loss of pigment, which manifests as white patches.

WHITEHEAD – forms when oil and dead cells accumulate and block the hair follicles.

XANTHELASMA – yellow patches that are usually found in the soft skin around the eyes and may be a result of fatty deposits.

ZYDERM – bovine collagen that is used to improve the appearance of wrinkles and scars, and to add volume to the lips.

ZYPLAST – cross-linked form of collagen also used to fill wrinkles and add volume to the lips.

Useful contacts

www.iranderma.com
Dermatological associations around the world

www.dermalinstitute.com
The International Dermal Institute

www.plasticsurgeons.co.za
Association of Plastic and Reconstructive Surgeons of Southern Africa

www.baps.co.uk
British Association of Plastic Surgeons

www.totalskincare.com
Skincare issues, treatments and advice

www.isaps.org
International Society of Aesthetic Plastic Surgery

www.surgery.org
The American Society for Aesthetic Plastic Surgery

www.dermatology.about.com
Collection of various articles, as well as product reviews and treatments for skin disorders

www.oneskin.com
All you need to know about skin ailments

Index

Bold entries indicate illustrations or photographs

Picture credits

All photographs for New Holland Publishing © Ian Reeves at Shine Group with the exception of the following photographers and/or their agents listed below: